DIGNIFYING DEMENTIA

A Caregiver's Struggle

ELIZABETH TIERNEY

Published by OAK TREE PRESS, 19 Rutland Street, Cork, Ireland
www.oaktreepress.com
www.dignifyingdementia.com

© 2011 Elizabeth Tierney

A catalogue record of this book is available from the British Library.

ISBN 978 1 904887 70 6 (ePub)
ISBN 978 1 904887 71 3 (Kindle)
ISBN 978 1 904887 72 0 (Paperback)
ISBN 978 1 904887 88 1 (Hardback)

This is a true story. However, the names and / or personal
details of some of the people mentioned have been changed
to protect their privacy.

CONTENTS

PROLOGUE

*The only kind of dignity which is genuine is
that which is not diminished by the
indifference of others.*

Dag Hammarskjöld

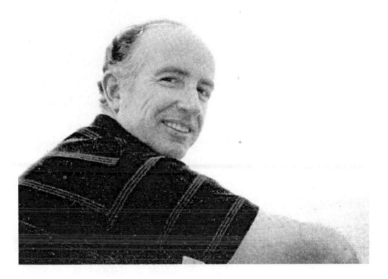

Diagnosed with dementia in 1997, my husband, Jim, lived at
home during his illness and died there in January 2006.

I wish this story were fiction, but it is not. Jim might have
considered my writing about him a betrayal, and 'betrayal' is the
word he would have used.

Far from a betrayal, this is both a love story and an attempt to
reach out to others who are living through or who will live

through a similar tragedy. It is written in the hope that others might benefit from what I learned as the caregiver of a dementia victim. Only then will Jim's cruel affliction serve some purpose, because it might help others feel less lonely, bewildered, angry or frustrated than I did, shorten the dreadful learning curve, or encourage others to ask more questions and make fewer assumptions. And because it might remind members of the health care industry – from physicians to orderlies, from agency administrators to certified nursing assistants – that dementia victims and their loved ones are human beings who deserve respect, kindness, empathy and patience, so often lost in our fast-paced society. The diagnostic process I describe was painful and disappointing; perhaps someone else's experience might be easier. Caring for Jim was exhausting; perhaps someone else's caregiving might be less draining. Losing Jim this way – incomprehensible. I offer no advice about repairing a broken heart. I can do nothing for mine.

During the years of Jim's illness, when I overheard people arguing over what to buy or where to eat or what store to go to, I wanted to walk over to them and say, "You are wasting precious time. You never know what might happen, what may be taken away." In fact, someone once said to me, "You must have just realized what you lost." No, happily and sadly, I knew.

Jim probably suffered from Lewy Body Dementia (LBD). Why 'probably'? Only an autopsy would have been definitive, but on the day he died, too stunned, I forgot to remind the funeral home to send his remains to the Alzheimer's Disease Research Center at Duke University.

Most people are probably more familiar with Alzheimer's Disease (AD) – as one aide called it, 'Old Timer's Disease' – and use that name for all dementias. Sadly, there are others. According to the Alzheimer's Association, 50% to 70% of dementias are Alzheimer's but there's also Parkinson's Disease with Dementia (PDD), Creutzfeldt-Jacob Dementia (CJD),

Normal Pressure Hydrocephalus (NPH) and Pick's Disease (PiD), to name a few.

They remind me of the initials of the Roosevelt years: SEC, TVA, FDIC – initials designed to make a country well, unlike these, which are destructive, heartrending initials for illnesses that steal the victims from the people who love them and from themselves. These illnesses are not 'long goodbyes'. That phrase is too genteel. Watching someone lose his or her mind and body is not polite. It is rude and mean-spirited. True, it can be 'long'; for us, it was almost a decade.

Tragically, these neurodegenerative illnesses affect many lives, and the number of dementia sufferers is expected to rise significantly over the coming decades – with no cure to date. In December 2005, *The Lancet* reported the findings of a major study indicating that, by 2040, the number of victims will be a staggering 81.1 million people, with a diagnosis every seven seconds. According to the 2010 *Alzheimer's Facts and Figures*, 5.3 million people in the United States have Alzheimer's. I remember a physician's saying, "People in nursing homes either have dementia or are about to get it." While these diseases are spoken about in terms of millions, they are about individuals, the victims themselves and the people who love them – the caregivers.

These diseases are heartless to victim and caregiver alike. I still see the terror in Jim's eyes when he didn't recognize me or his own surroundings, and I still feel the heartache when I could do nothing to help him. Dementia brutalized him and stole the love of my life from me. It altered him, us and me.

Jim was neither wealthy nor powerful; he was not an Alzheimer's sufferer like Ronald Reagan, Iris Murdoch, Charles Bronson, Sargent Shriver, Perry Como or Charlton Heston, nor a Parkinson's victim of the stature of Janet Reno, Michael J. Fox or John Lindsay. Jim's picture did not appear on the front page of

The Independent, The Times or *The New York Times* when he died. He was simply a gentle soul and a good man.

This book is divided into four sections. **Part One** describes our life together before Jim's illness and the first signs that all was not well. **Part Two** tells of our desperate search for a diagnosis and the beginning of his decline. **Part Three** speaks of his continuing deterioration and my acceptance that I needed help caring for him and the implications of that realization. **Part Four** is about the emotional and economic costs associated with his illness.

This is not a medical text; it is the story of our experience with dementia and the lessons I learned as I tried to be his voice, to maintain his dignity and to care for him and for me.

৩ ৫

> *A short winter this one,*
> *When all the joys of spring*
> *Conspire to lie about the season.*
>
> *Nothing here is real,*
> *Not snow, not cold,*
> *Not raw damp chill upon the heart;*
> *But the soft whisper*
> *And the private look,*
> *And the sweet touch of a gentle hand.*
>
> *A short winter, this one,*
> *To learn a rule of life:*
> *One must be content*
> *To be happy in small ways.*
>
> **Jim Tierney**

PART ONE

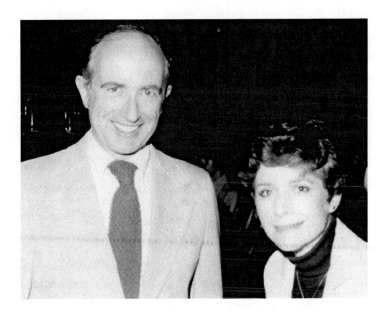

I lay in bed listening for the sound of Jim's breathing. Under the blanket his body was still. In the darkness, I couldn't see his chest moving, and in the silence I couldn't hear a sound. *Is he alive? Please, Love, please be alive. Oh, God, is he dead? Please, be gone. Then it'll be over. No! No, Cookie, please don't be dead, please.*

I inched up onto my left elbow, moved my right hand near his face where I thought his nose must be, took a deep breath, let it out and closed my eyes. I felt the warmth of his exhalation on my palm. *He's alive. Thank God! Thank God!* But, oh, it would be easier if he weren't breathing, if he were dead. Easier? No, I'm not sure, but the ordeal would be over – quietly and peacefully in his sleep.

Was Jim as ambivalent as I was about his dying? Was he even aware of life and death? 'Ambivalent'? What a word! The 4:00 or the 7:00 movie? Pizza or a sandwich? That's 'ambivalence.' Given Jim's demented condition, why, one might ask, would I want him to live or die? Because if he died, I would miss that miraculous smile, those laughing blue eyes, and the remnants of his speech, those once-a-day utterances – without context – when he was "leaving for Ireland with the President" or "going to teach me rugby." Why would I want him to die? Then this seemingly cell-by-cell death would be over, as would my standing by watching a vital person transformed into a drooling infant.

For nine years, we were in limbo. How had we come to this point?

৯৽ ৵৩

In the summer of 1997, I rushed Jim to the emergency room at our local hospital because he was bleeding rectally. A doctor took Jim's history and then asked to speak to me outside the cubicle where Jim was lying on a gurney. I am five feet tall. The emergency room doctor, a man over a foot taller, looked down at me and said, "Your husband has dementia." Without another word, he strode down the corridor. Dumbfounded, I watched him walk away and knew without a doubt that this guy was an idiot!

What did he mean Jim had dementia? What kind of diagnosis was that and on what did he base it? Nothing was wrong with Jim's mind! He spoke clearly. He responded to questions. Why? For heaven's sake, Jim was bleeding and scared. Because Jim turned to me for some of the details of his medical history?

Because he couldn't remember the date of the lithotripsy for his kidney stones? Was that why?

Jim could have cared less about medical details. In fact, he disliked dealing with medicine, and to Jim, doctors were the same as auto mechanics. They knew how the body worked, and you went to them to get the car or the body serviced or the part replaced. Being the medical historian was my job, not Jim's. It was part of our unofficial pre-nuptial agreement. I answered the phone, remembered birthdays and made the appointments with dentists, doctors, plumbers, electricians, friends and family.

Jim, on the other hand, cooked, vacuumed, washed the dishes, waxed the floors, and dumped the trash. He did the laundry. He made the bed in the morning, and if I ventured into his territory, he took the trash bag or vacuum out of my hand. Occasionally, I was permitted to cook.

Jim didn't have dementia. I knew what dementia was. I had seen the results of the scourge. My father was diagnosed with Parkinson's with Dementia and needed a 'minder' for years, until he was admitted to a nursing home because his violent outbursts became too much for my frail, osteoporotic, rheumatoid-arthritic mother. My dad, the surgeon, loved practicing medicine, solving crossword puzzles, reading, going to art museums, and walking his dog. My dad, who took up the flute in retirement, had been reduced to a shell of a man unable to talk, walk or see. I knew dementia destroys lives and homes, causes the normal to become abnormal and the abnormal the norm. Good grief, Jim was not demented. He had rectal bleeding!

ॐ ॐ

So besides our division of labor, who were we? We were simple folks, living uncomplicated lives. Jim was James, *Seamus* in Irish. His middle name was Benignus – for Brother Benignus, a local priest in Ireland. I am Elizabeth. Ours was a second marriage for both of us. He was a kind, unassuming man, who earned his living as a teacher and educational administrator. He was the funny, intelligent, hard-working, sensitive man I was fortunate enough to meet, fall in love with and with whom I spent half my life. I knew Jim for over 30 years and was married to him for 25.

A colleague introduced us. Jim was the Chairman of the English Department in a new high school in New York City. After six years at one school, I had become increasingly uncomfortable walking up and down the stairs with the kids and with the installation of a metal detector in the lobby. I saw a student carrying a gun at a dance, lost another who was killed after he made a winning basket at an after-school center and learned that yet another student missed classes because of the bullet wound in his leg. I was ready for a change.

The interview with Jim Tierney was scheduled for June 14, 1974. I remember the charm of the man; he remembered my red dress. A few weeks later, Jim called to offer me a job. I said, "Yes" and taught English in his department for four years, until I earned my doctorate and accepted my first supervisory position.

In late December 1974 we were chatting outside his office after school; the conversation became personal. He knew I was a single parent. "How come you never remarried?" he asked. "Because I never met anyone like you," I said. Silence. *Where did that come from?* I was trembling. We said, "Good night." I left. *What had I said!*

The next morning as I was punching in my time card, Jim put his head in the doorway of the front office, smiled and said, "I have made a decision." With those words, our love affair began.

Jim was married at the time, but once he announced that he had made a "decision," we met at a local diner where we talked for hours, or we sat and talked in a cold car in a parking lot. It wasn't until a grad school classmate of mine offered us her apartment that we became lovers.

The following spring Jim moved out of his house into his own apartment. He left with his clothes, a box of books, some photographs, some paintings and a mountain of guilt. Instead of having more time together, Jim distanced himself from me. He brooded, drank his Beefeater's Gin, cried, drank and cried. On some days he invited me to come over for a few minutes after school, but as the gin flowed, he said, "Go home." He was riddled with guilt, and I felt helpless as I watched him weep, drink and regret.

In our years together Jim never talked to me about his first marriage, but a few years ago, an old friend of Jim's said, "Jim's marriage had been over for years; he stayed until the kids were grown." I never heard Jim say that, but he was a fiercely private, decisive man who could say, "Let it go," and did, while I, the worrier, dwelled.

ço ۔ø

Jim mended slowly from leaving his marriage; we lived apart. However, when a school district offered me an administrative position, Jim said, "Let's live together." We did. Then, after Jim's divorce became final, we married in a judge's law office. Romantics that we were, we both had gone to work in the morning and celebrated by dining out that evening with Ellen, my daughter, the other important person in my life. Over the years we celebrated birthdays and anniversaries with dinner or lunch at a restaurant.

A sensitive soul with demons and self-doubts, Jim was a respected administrator, who worked hard and fostered loyalty. If school began at 8:30, Jim was there at 7:00. He served the teachers and the principal, who considered him his *consigliere*. Not only did Jim work long days, he also worked long weeks. When I met him, he had his day job, his night job and his weekend jobs – one at a Yeshiva – and when he quit the weekend job, he immediately became an adjunct instructor at a local college, where I taught also.

Jim cared about making a difference in education. One piece of advice he gave me when I stepped into my first administrative job was, "Do everything you can to help teachers improve, but be prepared to make a decision one way or the other the very first time you observe them."

He had a beautiful voice, was soft-spoken and mild-mannered. Only once do I recall his losing his temper at work. Those of us who heard his raised voice were stunned. Jim Tierney shouting? I mustered the courage to ask him what had happened. He winked at me. He said, "I wasn't angry. It was meant for everyone to hear." He grinned and said, "It's important that people think you're a little nuts." He was right. We all toed the line after that.

When I became a supervisor, college lecturer, assistant superintendent, trainer, writer, speaker, whatever, I turned to Jim to help solve problems, because his skills, gut, patience, good sense and wit were invaluable.

For example, in my new district, the superintendent delighted in using my shiny, new doctorate as a wedge among his other administrators. Divide and conquer, I supposed. Each quarter the superintendent evaluated us with a 'motivational document' he had developed. On each of over 200 items, he gave a 'C' for commendable, 'S' for satisfactory or 'N' for needs improvement. After each evaluation the administrators would gather and ask each other, "How many Cs did you get?" Jim had suggested that, after the evaluation, I innocently ask my colleagues, "How do you get Cs?" I did. Immediately, my colleagues became solicitous. With one strategic question, my guru had diffused the tension.

∽ ∾

While Jim had a Machiavellian, sardonic sense of humor, he was also a self-effacing loner, who frequently said, "I'm not good at small talk." Despite that opinion, people were struck by his intelligence, humor and enviable command of language. He had a mellifluous voice and a wonderful laugh. But he struggled with a sense of inadequacy. Believe it or not, he was loath to change a light bulb for fear of breaking it. He would ask me, half in jest, what I saw in him. He said, "I am an old man, and you are 16." Not quite, we were 10 years apart. I was 55 when he was first diagnosed with dementia; he was 65.

As for his physical health, nothing unusual, he struggled with high blood pressure, high cholesterol, kidney stones and, eventually, poor hearing. Ironically, once he became ill, his blood pressure was perfect.

His insecurity probably stemmed from his childhood, about which he often spoke. A Leo, he was born in the Bronx, New York, on August 19, 1932, of an Irish mother and father who had immigrated to the United States. According to her death certificate, his mother, Anna, died of a postpartum hemorrhage on the day of his birth – a fact that colored his life. His father returned to Ireland, and Jim was left in the care of his grandmother, who eventually brought the toddler back to Drimnagh, a working class neighborhood in Dublin, there to be reunited with his father – and his father's new wife.

Jim often said, "I felt I didn't belong to that family." When Jim was a young teenager, he found a Mass card with the name Anna Geary Tierney on it. Only when he confronted his father with it was he told of his mother's death and learned that his 'mother' was his stepmother and the other children, stepbrothers and stepsisters. Only then was he introduced to his mother's family in Aglish, County Waterford. When I met Jim, he spoke with affection of his Uncle Jack and seemed removed from the rest of his family – particularly his father.

According to Jim, his father was impatient and frustrated by Jim's lack of manual dexterity and by his love for books. A voracious reader, Jim talked of 'mitching' (cutting) from school, strolling along the used bookstalls by the River Liffey, or biking into the Dublin hills to read, or hiding under the covers at night with a book. Jim won a scholarship to the prestigious Synge Street School in Dublin, where, like his father, the Christian Brothers beat him.

Jim needed to read every day: newspapers, magazines and books. He read a daily paper, preferably *The New York Times* and, on Sundays, he savored his favorite section, the *Book Review*. Until the editorial changes, he looked forward to the arrival of *The New Yorker* and read it cover to cover and missed the *Saturday Review*. Jim's idea of a good time always included a book: Friel, Parker, Yeats, Wilde, O'Neill, Synge, Shaw, McDonagh, O'Faoláin, Higgins, Trevor, le Carré, Kinnell, and Ellman.

In time, Jim's father re-immigrated to the States with his family. Once again in New York City, Jim attended Power Memorial and went on to Fordham University. He worked; he studied; he married. He said to me, "I married in part to get away from my father." Jim had four children.

While he was in school, he had a part-time job at the now defunct men's clothing store, Rogers Peet. An Irish-Catholic in a predominantly Jewish business, he referred to himself as the "token goy." Clothing and appearance mattered to Jim, and Ireland and Rogers Peet influenced his style: herringbone tweeds, moleskin slacks, silk rep ties, Johnston Murphy shoes or his elegant Ferragamo loafers. An Irishman, he probably would have worn his Sunday best when he gardened if I hadn't introduced him to the notion of wearing blue jeans and Rockport sneakers.

ɢ ɞ

Rockport shoes and Rockport, Massachusetts – Jim loved the sea, to travel and have 'adventures.' With the extra money I earned from seminars based on my dissertation on the use of the novel in the training of managers, we rented a house in Rockport, Massachusetts for the summer. There, we walked along Marmion Way, along Back Beach into town, up to Bearskin Neck to look at the water, the lobstermen and their boats.

He also loved gentle hill country. One weekend we went to Berkshire County in Western Massachusetts. On the drive back to our rental apartment near the city, he suggested we consider buying a house in Columbia County in upstate New York – it reminded him of Ireland. And, he said, "A house would be a great tax write-off." Irishman that he was, Jim preferred owning rather than renting.

So, on another weekend, we went to look for a house. On the way, we played 'Which House Would YOU Buy.' Near the realtor's office, we saw a little white Cape sitting on about an acre of land. We both shouted, "That one!" We described the house to the realtor who said, "It's for sale and has a low bid on it." We looked at the house and made an offer: one afternoon, one house, one offer – a few phone calls later, a mortgage application, help from my dad, and we were homeowners.

We had a weekend house. There, our cat, Mulligan, roamed about the yard, stalked deer, caught garden snakes, brought field mice to the doorstep, pounced on falling leaves and was nearly savaged by an enraged blue jay.

Our neighbors, Peggy and John Simpson, were kind, generous and, unknowingly, anxiety-producing. If Jim saw John driving his tractor mower, Jim would laugh and say, "Oh, God, I have to get out there. I can't have our grass a quarter of an inch higher than John's." And off he would go to mow.

Jim planned and farmed a patch of land; he grew tomatoes, corn, grapes and asparagus. He plotted revenge on Japanese beetles, deer, woodchucks and rabbits. He cleared raspberry bushes and reclaimed land. Meanwhile, I worried about his blood pressure and overexertion, as I watched him pushing his mower up the back hill. He was delighted with the used, red Ariens tractor mower I bought him for his birthday.

In essence, life was easy. On Sunday mornings we headed to the Bakery for pancakes or French toast. When Jim wasn't mowing, raking, pruning or weeding, he was in the hammock reading a book or *The Sunday Times*. In the winter we read by the fire and walked in the snow.

Like most weekenders, we delighted in the scenery, the fresh air and the quiet. Soon, we decided to leave on Monday mornings at 4:00 am, rather than drive back to our apartment on Sunday afternoons. That way we had a few more hours in the country before heading back to work. Jim drove. I was the deer lookout, and the threat of a snowstorm didn't stop him from making that two hour and 10-minute drive each way every weekend. In all, we may have missed only one or two weekends a year.

ço ꜩ

Eventually, we thought about giving up our apartment near the city and living full-time in the country. To do that we needed jobs in the area. One Sunday we saw an ad for the English Chair at Hudson Valley Community College (HVCC) in Troy, New York, about 40 minutes north of our weekend home. We decided we would both apply for the position, and, if either of us got the job, we could become full-time residents. Amazingly, we were both called for interviews – on the same day – at 10:00 and 11:00. I went first, and on my way out I whispered to Jim, "It's your job. They have union troubles."

Jim had been the United Federation of Teachers' (UFT) chapter chairman before becoming an administrator. The selection committee at Hudson Valley Community College put three names before the board: Jim's, mine and that of a third candidate. We waited several months to hear the results. I was number two. They named Jim Chairman of the English Department.

Thus, our weekend house became our year-round home. Two years later when we were on vacation in Ireland, Jim called his secretary, Lorraine, from a phone booth on a windy Rosses Point in County Sligo. For an unassuming man with his own demons and insecurities, that call was special. Jim had applied for another position at the college. Lorraine told him that he had been named Dean of Liberal Arts and Sciences. He looked so proud and happy, and I was thrilled for him. To celebrate, he said, "Buy yourself a present."

"Get something for yourself," was typical of Jim. At times his reluctance to celebrate or buy gifts for me or for anyone else made me 'nuts.' I, on the other hand, loved to give him presents: books, pipes, trips, clothes and even tractor mowers. When it came to buying presents or to writing poetry, he had to be perfect – certainly never wanting. Would that he had written more.

His forgetting my 50th birthday was particularly painful. I remember looking at him just before I left for work, saying, "Would you please wish me a Happy Birthday?" He grimaced. Don't ask me how he managed it, but within minutes, I was feeling sorry for him because he was feeling guilty about having forgotten.

ɕ ᴥ

Even though I had applied for the chairman's job at HVCC, within three years of earning my PhD in education I wearied of the school business. I resigned my administrative position and took a job as a recruiter with a personnel agency in Manhattan.

Despite welcoming the change, I was terrified of leaving my job, my profession and working on commission.

My mother's reaction was, "What are you making? Nothing?"

Always my supporter, Jim said, "You're the gutsiest broad I know." And added, "Don't worry. We'll be fine."

He was right.

I enjoyed personnel work; it was fast-paced, required listening, planning, problem-solving, motivating, involved no committees, and I felt I had a more immediate impact on someone's life. But once Jim was working full-time at the college, I began looking for work upstate because the six-hour, round-trip, scenic commute into the city by car and rail was expensive and exhausting. In time we commuters came to know each other very well; we knew who slept, worked or chatted on the ride into Manhattan. We even organized a picnic for commuters and trainmen at Claremont Park. Around the holidays, regular passengers brought chocolate truffles and wine.

Occasionally I stayed over in our rental apartment near the city. Over the years Jim and I were rarely apart – so few times, in fact, that I can name them: obligatory work-related retreats and conferences – in Saratoga for Jim and Williamstown, Lakeville and Gettysburg for me; overnight hospital stays in Dublin, Hilton Head and Boston and Jim's trip to Ireland. We preferred each other's company.

Whenever we were apart, I phoned Jim to catch up on the day's events. One night he said, "The mosquitoes are merciless. I have been clearing the yard, and I'm covered with bites. Frankly, I'm not feeling well." The next day when I returned home, I saw that Jim's itch was not caused by insect bites. He had a rash from poison ivy. Mosquitoes? Poison ivy? What mattered to Jim was the bottom line – he itched.

After one awful 11-hour round-trip train ride, my half-hearted job search upstate became more aggressive. While I thoroughly enjoyed what I was doing in personnel, we weren't living in a 'wired' society yet, and the commuting was wearing.

We were able to let go of the apartment when I was hired as Personnel Director for an educational services organization about 35 minutes from home. The organization provided shared services to school districts. Along with my Human Resources duties, I had an opportunity to design handbooks, create a recruiting fair as well as several educational seminars for administrators.

One day, the superintendent of one of the participating districts spoke to me privately, "Would you be interested in the position of Assistant Superintendent in my district?" I said, "Yes." She added, "I am going to speak to your Superintendent and ask for you to apply," and she added, "And I want you to act surprised when he tells you." I said, "I will." Mistake! I should have consulted Jim.

A month or so went by, my boss called me into the office and told me about the position, and I did as I had promised – I acted surprised. I applied, was appointed and became operationally responsible for the district during a political 'mess.' We reopened the pool and the library, scheduled assemblies, put student artwork in the halls, organized a major outdoor event, hired new staff and encouraged team teaching. It was a great and gratifying challenge.

However, my former boss had a long memory and didn't forgive. He learned that I had known I was going to be recruited and was livid that I had been dishonest with him and had misplaced my loyalty. So when the Superintendent's position in the district became available, and the school board put my name forward, I was told that my previous boss told the school board in no uncertain terms that he would oppose my candidacy. While the board had given me authority and supported my recommendations for change in the district, they acceded to his position. No surprise. But I was devastated. After the initial shock, I began looking for jobs elsewhere. Jim came with me on the interviews. But I realized that, even though the names changed, the public school business was the same.

ℰ ℯ

One night we were home sitting by the fire. "Why don't we move to Ireland?" For years afterwards, we debated which of us had had the 'epiphany.' It was to become our final great adventure – and 'great' it was.

Why Ireland? When we first met, Jim talked of his 'love-hate' relationship with the country. In 1976, I bought him a present of a round-trip ticket for a two-week vacation during the Easter break. Tears came to his eyes when I surprised him with a model of an Aer Lingus plane and his ticket. He flew to Ireland, traveled around the country and saw his Uncle Jack for the last time.

Three years later Jim and I went on a two-week vacation to Ireland – my first trip. I loved the country, the blue and gray skies, the openness and warmth of the people, the lush countryside. We saved our money and our vacation days and went to Ireland for our annual two-week vacations as often as we could. One year on the way to the airport, I gave Jim a gold self-winding watch for his birthday.

Our half-joke about relocating to Ireland became a reality. Even though his pension was small, Jim was old enough to retire and did, and he was champing at the bit to leave. I, however, needed a few more weeks at work to ensure my pension rights. When I gave notice, we put our house and car on the market, arranged for the driveway to be plowed and for friends to watch the house. Sadly our cat, Mulligan, had disappeared one night. We arranged for our new cat, Molly, to be adopted by a friend –

who promptly flew with her to St. Thomas in the Virgin Islands. Over the years, we had Daedalus, Blazes, Mulligan and Molly – all Joycean cats. Guess who named them?

As eager as I was to try our six-month 'adventure,' I felt guilty leaving my aging parents and my daughter Ellen, who was now living in New York after having graduated from Vassar. I remembered justifying the decision by saying, "We have to do this now, because you never know what's going to happen."

ও ৫

We flew to Ireland in January 1989. The daffodils were blooming when we landed in the morning in a frosty Dublin. We had our savings – $10,000 – and planned to try three months on the east coast of Ireland and three on the west. Jim's new pension just covered our expenses at home: car payments, mortgage, utilities and snowplowing. I had no income. We spent the first night in Dublin in a 'grotty,' cold bed and breakfast, wondering what the hell we had been thinking.

Very quickly we learned that there wasn't a job to be had and that we could only rent for a minimum of six months, so we decided to try Dublin for the six months. Naturally rents for our first flat were higher than we wanted to pay, and the rate of exchange was not in our favor. While I was quietly freaking out, Jim said, "Have faith. Things work out." They did. Our six-month experiment lasted six years.

We took a taxi to our first flat in Dublin. The next year we drove our leased Mini to our new rental cottage in a village further south in County Wicklow. A year later we needed several trips in our leased four-door car for our third move to a mews house, also in County Wicklow. We were acquiring 'stuff' – our boxes of clothes, books, LPs, and pictures that we had packed before we left – ready for shipping.

We had spent most of our $10,000 by the time our car sold in the States. The very next week I came back home with my first IR£200 check. I had been paid for consulting on a PriceWaterhouse/University College Dublin (UCD)/Hungarian Ministry of Agriculture project. Really! That 'gig' led to a lectureship and process consultancy on the Faculty of Commerce at UCD. I taught graduates, undergraduates, and postgraduates, and the dean asked me to develop courses in Business Ethics as well as Personal Skills in Business. I even taught in Hungary.

Soon, in addition to the lecturing and consulting work at UCD, I was delivering workshops for the Irish Sate agency for hospitality and management seminars for a British training company. I wrote seven 'how-to' books, as well as academic and popular articles for journals, magazines and papers. I spoke at conferences in Killarney, Waterford and Belfast. What a life! It was unbelievable!

One afternoon Jim said, "You owe your former boss a thank you." What? I couldn't believe my ears. I was still smarting from the blow to my career and my ego. Jim said, "He did you a big favor. If it hadn't been for him, you'd still be there!" Right again, Jim. He turned my simmering anger into gratitude.

Our lives were idyllic. We strolled along the strand, along the piers at Dun Laoghaire. One evening, we were delighted by a window in a bookshop downtown; it was covered with posters promoting my first book, *ShowTime!* We visited Jim's old neighborhoods in Dublin. We drove through the mists of Connemara and walked around Galway. We meandered through Cork, Waterford and Portumna. We went to see the Druid Theatre Company, and to the Gate and the Abbey Theatres. We ate fresh scones and jam in Enniskerry.

Jim drank Jameson in the pubs in Dublin; we ate sausages at Bewley's. We walked. We laughed. We had cold feet and noses at night. Jim bought treats for Kelly, the golden retriever, who visited the mews house. Our biggest problems required Jim to shoo sheep off the front lawn, get mice out of the cabinets, or ask the traveling people, the tinkers, to leave the property. One morning as I was driving to work, two horses galloped down a hill into the side of our car. Neither of the horses was hurt, nor was I, and no one at UCD was remotely taken aback by my excuse for being late.

While Jim welcomed retirement and chose not to work, he did write some articles for *Variety International*. Always introspective, the interviewing process made him uncomfortable, and he no longer wanted responsibility. He wanted to read, to walk and to travel.

Eventually, our little house in upstate New York sold. I felt sad. But ever the pragmatist, Jim said, "It was time to sell it. I was worried about the plumbing."

With Jim's pension, my income from the university and no more financial responsibilities in the States, we were able to travel. I was always a nervous flyer, so Jim held my hand on every flight, but he insisted on my looking out the window at the sights as the plane banked to the right or left. We traveled together to conferences in London, Bath, Luxembourg and Milan and to deliver training courses in Manchester, Budapest, Belfast and Debrecen.

And for pure fun, we visited Rimini, Florence, Copenhagen, Bruges, Athens, Palma, Amsterdam, Moscow, St Petersburg, Helsinki, Oslo, Warsaw, Berlin, Paris, Cannes and Monaco. We stared in disbelief at the Kremlin, Checkpoint Charlie, St Peter's and Elsinore. We held hands wherever we went. We ate thin-crusted pizza in Nice, ordered *moules avec pommes frites* in Bruxelles, ate croissants in Paris. We fought off urchins in Rome and got caught in a train strike in Sorrento and a vaporetto strike in Venice.

And always, in addition to the museums and palaces, bookstores were part of the itinerary. Jim could sniff out

bookstores in Europe as well as he had in the States. He went to
the Strand or the Gotham in New York, Toad Hall in Rockport,
Shaver's in Savannah, the Harvard Book Store in Cambridge. In
Europe there was Shakespeare and Company in Paris,
Waterstone's and Hatchard's in London, Kenny's in Galway,
Hodges Figgis in Dublin. He didn't necessarily buy; he browsed.
However, he would buy Bernard McLaverty, Desmond Hogan,
Michael O'Siadhail, Lar Redmond, Bernard Farrell and add
them to his "Irish collection." Books were always in his life. He
once said, "It's time to get rid of the books." I couldn't. We
didn't. They traveled with us.

ം~ ~ം

Even in the south of France, Jim found English books. During
UCD's winter semester break we headed to Nice, because we
enjoyed the food, the open markets, the sunshine and the walk
along the *Promenade des Anglais*, where we admired the elegant,
mink-clad women walking their equally fashionable, adored,
adoring and adorable dogs.

One winter, though, our travel agent in Ireland said that the
studio apartment we had previously rented in Nice was
unavailable. I was disappointed. "What if we go to Hilton Head,
South Carolina instead? It's off-season," I said. "We would be
paying for the trip in Irish punts, and with the rate of exchange
in our favor, we could afford to go. And the water pressure
would be a refreshing change." Hilton Head came to mind
because we had spent a pleasant week's vacation there some
years earlier and had returned for a conference, where
serendipitously an editor bought the rights to *ShowTime!*, which
was added to their academic series. The magic seemed to be
non-stop.

Jim concurred. So that year over the winter holiday, we flew
to Hilton Head. We walked along the beach and biked the trails.

What do non-golfers do on rainy days? Look at real estate, of course. I asked Jim what he thought about buying a condo in Hilton Head. "If we owned a place, we could come to Hilton Head in the winter instead of worrying about whether we could get a studio in the south of France." We were renting in Ireland and no longer owned property, so I used his old line on him: "We would have a tax break." We bought a condo.

Shortly after returning to Ireland and to my classes at UCD, we received a phone call from my mother's live-in aide. Mom had been taken to the hospital diagnosed with a stroke; the physicians found breast cancer, too. We stayed in touch with her doctor and decided to fly back to New York to be with her. From there we returned to Hilton Head, found a nursing home and hired an air ambulance to fly her south. She died two weeks later. My profoundly demented dad was unaware of my mother's death. He died two years later – four months after Jim's initial diagnosis of dementia in June.

Earlier that year, as we had been walking along the strand in Bray, Jim had said, "It's time to go home." Did Jim have intimations of his own illness? How long after a neurodegenerative disease begins to wreak havoc before symptoms appear?

Leaving Ireland was bittersweet. Besides having fallen in love with the country, I was thriving on the lecturing, writing, speaking and consulting. Leaving brought it all to a sudden and dramatic halt.

≈

We were living in our condo in Hilton Head when Jim developed rectal bleeding. It was in South Carolina that the emergency room doctor said Jim had 'dementia' and walked away. Jim was admitted to the hospital, where a gastroenterologist treated him. An endoscopy revealed that Jim had a bleeding duodenal ulcer, which was repaired. After the procedure, the surgeon said to me, "Be sure Jim is never treated with Versed again." Versed is often used in surgery because it causes drowsiness, reduces anxiety and prevents memory of the event. The doctor said, "Instead of sedating him, the drug made him combative." Jim stayed overnight in the hospital – a night apart.

I went home and slept poorly, concerned not only about Jim's procedure but also about the offhand (but sadly accurate) remark about Jim's having dementia. I saw the image of my father in the nursing home – twisted, sightless and voiceless.

No, this could not be happening to my husband, too. Again, I asked myself, "What made the doctor say that?" He didn't know Jim. I calmed myself by repeating a phrase my statistics professor had used in grad school. This doctor was definitely "generalizing beyond his data."

Jim had never been the detail guy. Jim was the global member of our team. We had joked that he saw the 'forest for the trees,' and I saw the 'trees for the forest.' Jim wanted to buy the weekend house, to work upstate, to go to Ireland – the big picture. It was my job to implement the concept – his vision. That was not dementia; that was intuition and insight. He was the one who saw people for what they were, the one who said, "Why are you getting upset? You know who they are." Because Jim didn't remember dates, treatments or hospital stays? That wasn't dementia; that was lack of interest – like the itch he thought was from mosquitoes rather than from poison ivy. My dad referred to all birds as 'robins' and all flowers as 'roses.' I prayed, *Please, oh, please, let it be lack of interest.*

When I returned to the hospital in the morning, our regular internist was making his rounds and writing his notes. My eyes were brimming with tears of rage and frustration. I interrupted him as he was completing his paperwork and told him what the emergency room doctor had said to me about Jim's having dementia. Our internist looked up and said, "How does he handle the checkbook?" "How does he handle the checkbook? I do the checkbook," I said. "Just watch him," he said. That was that.

That June day was my personal 9/11. It was to become my first day as caregiver and bystander. I use the word 'bystander' deliberately; a doctor once referred to caregivers of dementia patients as bystanders because we are helpless.

I now know two kinds of helpless: 'helpless' being unable to talk to someone who is unhappy and 'helpless' watching someone's mind and body deteriorate from an incurable illness. I prefer the former. If you can communicate, there is hope. Profoundly depressed after the end of his marriage, Jim eventually rallied. Once he was ill, however, there was no hope. We could not change the course of the disease.

It also was the first day of my newfound contempt for, and distrust of, many members of the medical establishment. In time we would learn that the preliminary diagnosis was accurate, however reprehensible the manner of utterance. I felt both physicians lacked empathy for me and for Jim. They labeled, made short shrift of us and left.

Jim was discharged from the hospital with an admonition that the combination of taking daily baby aspirin and drinking alcohol causes gastrointestinal bleeding in some people. The good news was that Jim mended quickly.

The bad news was that I became hypervigilant and began watching Jim's every move. What I saw, or imagined I saw, was a man less inclined to make decisions, which frustrated me because I had delighted in his decisiveness. The man I had leaned on for quick answers seemed to be offering fewer, and I found myself agonizing over the wisdom of each one of mine. I remember and regret saying to him, "I feel as if I am leading two lives." Even going out to lunch became more difficult. He was passive. He would look at the menu and say, "Sweetie, I don't know what to get. You order." When the bill came, he would pull out his credit card from his wallet, hand it to me and say, "I'm buying. You add the tip and total it."

Not only was he becoming more indecisive, he was also becoming more insecure behind the wheel of the car. He had a panic attack driving over the Broad River Bridge. To me a panic attack crossing a bridge was understandable. I hate airplanes, suspension bridges and heights in general; the bridge was just under two miles long and only two lanes wide at the time. What was different was that Jim was the one having the panic attack – the man who held my hand on airplanes, the man who could deplane after a transatlantic flight at dawn – jetlagged – and drive the 135 miles from Shannon to Dublin in a stick-shift rental car on the left side of the road without missing a beat. This was the man who raced ahead of snowstorms, who drove to our weekend home year in and year out. The panic attack bewildered him, too. Unnerved, he asked me to drive back across the bridge.

Several times after that experience, he got behind the wheel of the car, drove a short distance and said, "I'm not feeling great. Do you mind driving?" He pulled over, walked around to the passenger side, while I got behind the wheel. The few times he did drive after that, I watched him grip the wheel with both hands, hug the curb, and drive well below the speed limit.

When he was driving, I noticed a faint tremor in the index finger of his right hand as it rested on the steering wheel. I drew it to Jim's attention. He dismissed it with, "It's probably the wheel alignment." A month or so later, he stopped driving altogether.

His walking changed too. In the past, whenever we walked, and I dragged my heels, he would look back at me and say, "Step it out." I had been hard pressed to keep up with him, but now he was keeping up with me.

He also told me that the self-winding watch I had given him years before was losing time or stopping. I suggested that, after all these years, it probably needed a good cleaning. Even after the repair, however, it still stopped, so we took it back to the jeweler.

The watch doctor said, "Are you swinging your arms? I have a client with Parkinson's whose watch doesn't work." I began to watch Jim's arms. He wasn't swinging them as he walked; they were hanging straight down and closer to his sides. We bought a $30 Timex.

In the first year after the casual emergency room diagnosis, Jim gave up driving, developed a tremor in his finger and became indecisive and withdrawn. While Jim had always preferred his own company and mine to the company of others, he occasionally welcomed joining friends for lunch or for a drink. Now he seemed to be avoiding other people, to be losing what confidence he had.

He also expressed concern about having difficulty concentrating on his reading. Not that! How many times over the years had he smiled and said, "I haven't read for two days. Would you go into town or have coffee with a friend, so I can read?" The last fiction he read was Richard Yates' *Collected Stories*; the last poets, Galway Kinnell, Paul Muldoon and Stanley Kunitz.

The healthy Jim enjoyed gardening, walking, traveling, smoking his pipe, drinking his Beefeater's Gin or glass of single malt, going to movies, watching *The Sopranos*, the Master's, the last game of the World Series, Wimbledon, March Madness and the World Cup. He ordered shrimp with hot garlic sauce, calamari in red sauce, trout amandine, pizza with *frutti di mare* with a half-bottle of wine. He preferred Monet and Van Gogh, listened to *Jacques Loussier Plays Bach*, Vivaldi, Britten, Mahler, Telemann, Delius and Herbie Hancock.

He loved to say, "It's you and me, kid." All too soon, it would become "You and me, kid, and dementia."

PART TWO

His tears began to flow. It was a secret river
that broke through all the dams. The river of
pain that everyone carried inside.

Henning Mankell

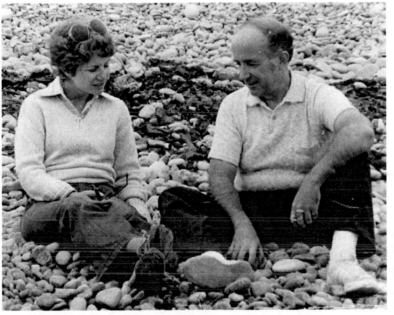

Photo: Ellen Graham

Living in Hilton Head meant we could take advantage of the mild, snowless days of winter. Our routine included arduous activities like walking on the beach, shopping for groceries, going to movies on Friday afternoons, keeping appointments with dentists or doctors, attending performances of the local theatres and orchestra and going out for lunch. Jim read. And we watched reruns of *Law and Order*. While Jim was more passive and wanted me to drive, nothing else in his behavior was shocking. Although he did have that disturbing little tremor.

Because of the internist's admonition about the checkbook, I watched Jim, and believing he could get better, I bought into the 'use it or lose it' notion. But when I encouraged or 'nagged' him to write or sign checks or add items to the grocery list, tears came to his eyes. When I bought a Scrabble set, he didn't want to play more than a game or two. When I asked him to edit a draft of something I had written, the process was painstaking for him, but I assumed it was either the content or my writing style causing the discomfort.

It's important to understand that living in Hilton Head violated one of Jim's few cardinal rules, which was: "We need to live within 100 miles of a major city." When we first moved to Hilton Head, we made excursions to Charleston, Gainesville, Atlanta, Jacksonville, St. Augustine, Aiken, Chapel Hill, Winter Park and Orlando in search of major cities and realized what we had done; we were living near charming, delightful 'towns,' not 'major cities.'

We knew we needed to spend part of every year near New York City. Like other snowbirds, we would migrate north when the snow melted to avoid the oppressive heat, humidity, mosquitoes and potential for hurricanes and to get a culture 'fix' to last us through the winter. We bought a tiny *pied-à-terre* half an hour from Manhattan and hired our first ever interior decorator. We dreamed, planned and behaved as if our lives were normal. We spent the summer inhaling the culture and then drove south for the winter filling our days with more walks, more movies and more mild days.

Come spring we headed north again. Once there in our little kitchen, we selected our adventures from the *Arts and Leisure*

section of the Sunday *New York Times*. We went to New York
Philharmonic rehearsals, concerts at Alice Tully Hall and at the
Merkin. We went to on, off and off-off Broadway Shows. We
saw foreign films in town, went to MoMA and the Metropolitan.
We discovered the Jupiter Symphony Chamber Players. And, of
course, every trip into the city included a visit to a bookstore. We
also saw our families.

Two years after the pronouncement by the ER doc, Jim was
having difficulty finding the precise word he wanted to use, no
longer drove and walked more slowly, but he did walk, and he
climbed onto buses and trains. At home he did the laundry,
made the bed, put groceries away, folded towels, read the paper,
used the remote control and went for strolls. Always a restless
soul, the notion of retiring was sitting badly with me; I wanted
to find a part-time job in the city for the following summer, and
happily I did.

෨ ෧

Amazingly, a friend of a high school classmate of mine called
and said he was looking for a pair of hands to help organize an
extra conference for his conference group. I was delighted to
have a three-day-a-week job in the city. I loved the work, the
people and being in town. On some weekends, we drove up to
the Berkshires to hear the Boston Symphony at Tanglewood.
When I was at work, Jim did what he loved to do: read, clean,
walk and read some more – although he repeated, "It's harder to
concentrate."

But all was not well. Not only was Jim having difficulty
finding the right word, he also was having difficulty
remembering and processing information. We had planned to
meet for lunch in town, when Jim phoned me at the office and
asked, "Which train ticket do I need to use to come into town?
Which one do I need for the return trip?" He could not

remember which of the two tickets lying side-by-side on the kitchen counter was for the train into town and which was the one for returning. We had talked about the tickets several times. I had even marked the full-fare and the off-peak tickets for him. He seemed unable to grasp the difference between the two.

That he phoned was remarkable. I was taken aback because he had always avoided using the telephone. Apparently the ticket problem was sufficiently important for him to make a call. While he sounded calm, I was not. When I hung up, after explaining once again which ticket to use for each trip, I should have reveled in the fact that he knew how to dial and get the answer to his question; instead, I was weeping.

I couldn't deny it any longer. Something WAS very wrong with Jim. He was unable to retain information and avoided interaction with people other than me. He asked me to buy train tickets for him and to talk to the stationmaster. If we took the train together, he handed me the tickets to give to the conductor. I bought the movie tickets. I asked for programs from the ushers, for the location of the men's room. He avoided talking.

Jim was losing control and his sense of humor.

Not long after he telephoned me about the train tickets, he took a phone message at home and made an error. In all the years I had known Jim, I couldn't recall his making any error when it came to words – ever. I had turned to him for spelling corrections, for grammar, for missing antecedents and misplaced modifiers. If he was unsure, he reached for our *Oxford Dictionary* in Ireland or for *Webster's* in the United States. He was my editor. He had written the phone message on a yellow post-it. It said, "Stephen called." As I read it, the breath went out of me. The man with the beautiful, open script had printed in large block letters, "Stephen called." The 'n' was backwards.

✎ ✎

Despite his withdrawal, his 'error' and word-finding problems, we continued our cultural spree.

One Saturday, we had tickets to a matinee at the Irish Repertory Company on 22nd Street. Jim, keeper of our theatre tickets, always put each set in a separate envelope with the show, theatre, address, time and date written on the front. On the day of the performance, he would transfer the tickets from the envelope to his wallet.

When I ordered these tickets, though, I said we would pick them up at the box office. The plan was to take the train into town, have lunch at a restaurant near the theatre, see the show, visit a bookstore, of course, and return home.

As planned, we took the train into Grand Central. While neither of us was particularly fond of subways, now that I was commuting, I had become cocky and convinced Jim that it was quicker to hop on the Lexington Avenue subway, get off at 23rd Street, walk west, have a leisurely lunch and take the heftier walk on our return to Grand Central after the show.

We arrived in town, walked to the subway entrance and took the escalator down to the platform. Our train was sitting in the station. I accelerated and stepped onto the car. The doors closed behind me. Jim was left standing on the platform as the train pulled out.

I pounded in vain on the doors and stood helplessly watching him through the glass. The woman beside me said, "My greatest nightmare is having the train door close before my daughter and I are both on or off the train together." I had never thought about it. I tried to remain calm and rational. Clearly, I had less confidence in Jim's ability to problem solve. What if he didn't remember where we were going? He had no tickets in his wallet. Why had I asked the theatre to hold our tickets at the box office? Why didn't we have a contingency plan?

I got off the train at 23rd Street and waited on the platform for the next southbound train. I watched the doors open, hoping I would see Jim get off the train. He didn't. The train pulled out. I waited for one more. No Jim. Then I raced upstairs to the street, hailed a cab and asked the driver to take me to Grand Central.

In the taxi, I visualized Jim walking upstairs from the subway to the information booth on the upper level. When I arrived, I paid the driver and ran from the cab into the 42nd Street entrance of Grand Central to retrace our steps. He wasn't at the information booth. I rushed back down to the subway platform. He wasn't there either, so I went back up to the information booth and asked to have him paged. They did. I waited. He didn't answer the page.

I replayed our conversation about going to the restaurant. Although we had never eaten there, I hoped he might remember the name, the location and walk to it. So I ran out of the station, grabbed another cab, this time back downtown to 22nd Street.

When I told the cab driver what had happened, he asked, "Why don't you have cell phones?" How sensible! We didn't. But what were the odds of Jim using one? Jim didn't like phones period, and he was uncomfortable with technology. My daughter had sent us her old computer, and I had prevailed on him to read an email or to look at *The Irish Times* online. He would humor me for a few minutes and then ask me to print out the article; he preferred the feel of paper in his hands. He considered himself a Luddite. Owning a cell phone had never occurred to me.

I hurried into the restaurant and looked around. No Jim. I asked the *maitre d'* if he would keep an eye out for a man about 5'7" in a black-and-white herringbone sports jacket. Then I rushed down the block to the theatre. It was around noon; the show started at 3:00. I waited. I paced. I walked back to the restaurant. I walked back to the theatre. Charlotte Moore, the Artistic Director of the Rep, asked how she could help; the waiters at the restaurant offered me coffee. Charlotte let me use the phone. I called Grand Central. I checked my timetable. I called home and left a message on the voicemail on the off-chance that Jim said, "Screw it" and returned home. Could he find his way home? I called home again. No answer. What were the odds of his accessing the voicemail, even though the directions and password were on a card by the phone?

I paced uselessly and explained to a woman waiting in the lobby that my husband had some memory problems. She said, "My husband had Alzheimer's. He died." I expressed my sympathy and knew her husband's problem had nothing to do with Jim's.

Time passed, no Jim. Charlotte said, "Perhaps he might have gone to the Irish Arts Center in midtown." Had Jim taken a train to Queens or Brooklyn? Was he at a police station? Was he wandering around lost? Had he been mugged? What must he be feeling? Does he know his New York address? He has his South Carolina driver's license. I said to myself, "Go home … no, stay."

At 2:55, as I was about to leave, and the curtain about to go up, Charlotte said, 'He's here." She had walked down the street and recognized the man I had described. She had said, "Jim?" He said, "Yes." He was there, really there. When he walked in, I hugged him. He felt sweaty through his wool jacket, and we hugged each other as if we had been separated for months.

I was so relieved to see him. We held hands. Charlotte offered us sodas and cookies and asked if we wanted to come back another day. We looked at each other and shook our heads, "No". She held the curtain for a few minutes and returned our ticket money. I lost a few months of my life that afternoon and felt indebted to all those New Yorkers.

I was beside myself that day because I was beginning to doubt his abilities. I should have had more faith in him. Apparently, when my train pulled out, he had taken the next one, a local, had gotten off at Astor Place and walked to the Public Theater. At the box office he asked if they were producing an Irish play. When he was told "No," he found a Barnes &

Noble and bought a copy of *The New Yorker*. He looked for the list of shows and particularly for ones with Irish names; then he walked to the Rep. He was holding the rolled up magazine when he arrived. He had needed to speak to only one person. Piece of cake! Why was I worried? Clearly, I was overreacting.

Despite that dramatic afternoon, we continued going to the theatre in the city – more often by car. I drove. On the weekends we drove up to Tanglewood to hear concerts conducted by James Conlon, Robert Spano, or Seiji Ozawa.

Jim struggled to find the right word and avoided conversations, but he still walked to the library and read. He bought groceries. He walked along the paths near the Parkway. He knew how to get home, to unlock a door, to make himself lunch. True, he was walking more slowly and having some 'memory problems.' If only his phone call to me about the train tickets, the message on the yellow post-it and the trip into town hadn't scared me so much.

During the previous winter, we had changed doctors in South Carolina. At our first meeting with our new internist, Jim had complained about not being able to concentrate. At the time, I had gotten testy when the doctor said, "Let's rule out Alzheimer's." But now, I was unsettled, so I phoned him to express my concern. "Enjoy the summer," he said, "we'll look at the problem when you return in the fall." Because he sounded calm, I tried to be too – sort of.

৵ ৵

Fall came. We packed, and I began the 800-mile drive south. Once on the road, though, I was on edge because I realized how vulnerable Jim was. True, Jim had found the theatre, but if I fell ill or 'dropped dead,' Jim would be in trouble. Thanks to the taxi driver's advice, I had a cell phone plugged into the console of the car for emergency use and had tried to show Jim how to press the buttons, but he had no interest in it or couldn't learn how to make it work.

Despite my anxiety, the drive was uneventful. We stopped at Hershey, Pennsylvania for the night and stayed at The Hotel Hershey – only the best for my mildly impaired Jim. I told myself to breathe and not to overreact. In fact, the next day, Jim helped navigate around the Beltway in DC – no easy feat under any circumstances.

When we arrived in Hilton Head, my neck and shoulder muscles were tight, and I woke up in the middle of the night with my heart racing, and I was sweating. I was scared. I didn't want to wake Jim, but I called 911 – something I had never done before.

The emergency medical technicians (EMTs) took my blood pressure and explained that I was OK but asked if I wanted to go to the hospital. I said, "My husband isn't well." Jim had slept through their arrival. They left, but I was still in a panic. I woke him and asked him to come to the hospital with me. Irresponsibly, I drove us to the hospital. My heart was OK, but my anxiety level was increasing; our internist gave me a monitor to wear. My fear was no longer just about flying and heights; it was now also about how Jim would manage if something happened to me.

Shortly thereafter, I met a woman who was asking herself the same question. What would happen to her husband if she died? Her husband had been diagnosed with Lewy Body Dementia and she with cancer. I had had the same fear as a single parent when Ellen was little; she, however, was adorable and had healthy grandparents.

※ ※

It was only a matter of days after returning to Hilton Head before the next distressing event happened. I had thought that the note on the yellow post-it was bad. Jim awakened and apologized for leaving his new clothes at Paul Stuart in New York. I showed him that they were in the closet and assumed he had had a dream.

A few days later, however, Jim woke up, sat up in bed, looked at me, smiled and said sweetly, "Where's your mother?" He asked me just like that. I didn't understand his question. I didn't know how to answer. Bewildered, I said, "Mom is dead." He asked again, "Where's your mother?" He was calm. I was, too. Was he dreaming? He climbed out of bed, took my hand and walked to the kitchen. He pointed to my handbag sitting on the kitchen counter and said, "Where is she?" I was dumbfounded and horrified. I said, "Sweetie, that's MY bag." Jim was looking for me.

Within five or 10 minutes, he was fine, and I was "Elizabeth" again. We sat down on the sofa. He said he felt a little heavy-headed and had no recollection of what had happened. I called our internist, who saw Jim that morning. After examining him, he said, "I am going to refer you to a neurologist, so we can rule out Transitory Ischemic Attacks (TIAs), mini-strokes." Aaah, 'to rule out.' Soon, I would wish that doctors could 'rule in.'

At our appointment, the neurologist asked Jim to count backwards by threes and to name the presidents in reverse order. That presidential question bothered me. I wanted to say, "We have been living in Ireland; ask him the names of the Irish or British prime ministers." I refrained. He also asked Jim to draw some diagrams, which he did with difficulty. Then the doctor recommended that Jim have a magnetic resonance imaging (MRI) scan.

We returned to the neurologist's office for the results of the MRI. The doctor slapped the films against the light box and said, "This is brain shrinkage, and I am 90% sure you have Alzheimer's." After that announcement, I tried to listen to his description of Jim's shrinking brain, but I stopped hearing and asking. I should have said, "What does brain shrinkage mean?" I should have said, "What about the TIAs? What does 90% sure mean?" I didn't. The doctor never looked at or spoke to Jim again, except when Jim asked quietly, "Do I need a home?" The neurologist said, "Why do you ask that?" and continued describing to me what he saw on the images – too much science.

He wrote a prescription for Zoloft to alleviate depression and Aricept to slow the progression of memory loss and told us to come back in three months. He recommended that Jim see a local psychologist for testing. Then he shook our hands, smiled and said, "Have a Merry Christmas!" He added happily, "I'm taking my family to Disney World." Like a robot, I said I was happy for him and wished him a Merry Christmas. I was numb. What had Jim comprehended? What were the implications of what we had been told? The doctor was only 90% sure, and we had a prescription for two drugs.

We had an emergency room doctor saying "Dementia," our internist saying "Let's rule out TIAs," and a "90% Alzheimer's" diagnosis from the neurologist. Could this be true? Didn't everyone's brain shrink with age? Maybe, oh maybe, the psychologist would be able to shed some light on what was happening.

That night when we climbed into bed, I hugged Jim and wept. He said, "Don't worry, kid. We'll get through it."

✎ ✎

Jim never liked tests, quiz shows, puzzles, card games or filling out applications. I had tried to twist his arm to play Scrabble. From time to time, I could get an answer to a crossword puzzle query. As for therapy, Jim accepted other people's seeing psychologists and psychiatrists, but he saw therapists as pseudo-priests who listened to confessions. However, in an effort to get more answers, and still believing we would, we followed up with the psychologist. Given his antipathy for short answer quizzes, I wondered how he would handle a 'battery of tests.' Wasn't it humiliating enough to be asked to count back from 100 by threes? He was willing to go. I prayed we would learn more.

The entryway to the psychologist's office was the first challenge. We looked at each other as we tried to figure out whether the door opened into a waiting room or into a private office. Finally, Jim knocked. The psychologist opened the door. Jim said, "I didn't know what to do, so I knocked." "Well, that's one way to handle it," the psychologist said. *Oh God, we are part of a 'door-opening' experiment.* Not an auspicious start.

The psychologist offered us chairs but never smiled. He asked Jim questions about his personal and professional life; then he took him into another room to give him some standardized tests. I couldn't believe how unfriendly he seemed. How was Jim going to relax? Afterwards the psychologist wrote a lengthy report indicating that there were "lapses in Jim's memory." Thanks! Didn't we know that without putting him through hoops? But we were no closer to knowing what was wrong, because rather than confirming that Jim had Alzheimer's, the psychologist wrote that the "lapses" or "cognitive impairment didn't appear to be Alzheimer's." Brain shrinkage? Didn't appear to be Alzheimer's? I, of course, held onto the phrase, 'lapses in memory.' But other than giving him humiliating tests and offering him drugs, why couldn't anyone tell us what was the matter with Jim? I was used to doctors being kind and definitive.

Winters had always included medical appointments, so in addition to seeing the neurologist and psychologist, Jim had an appointment with his urologist for a routine PSA (prostate-specific antigen) test to screen for prostate cancer. Jim's previous numbers had been elevated, and this test indicated that they still were, so the urologist recommended that Jim have a biopsy to determine whether there were any cancer cells. In preparation

Jim took Cipro, an antibiotic. He was accumulating prescriptions. The Aricept and Zoloft hadn't gone down well, so Versed was no longer the only culprit.

At 7:30 pm on December 31, 1999, New Year's Eve – Millennium Eve – Y2K Eve, the phone rang. I picked it up. It was the urologist. I signaled Jim. He picked up the extension. Jim asked me to stay on the line. The urologist said, "I wanted you to know that there are cancer cells in several quadrants of your prostate, and it's very treatable." He went on to explain radioactive seed implants. I could see Jim's face. After the opening remarks, he wasn't listening, just like me in the neurologist's office. Jim thanked the doctor for the call. But before we hung up, I blurted out, "By the way, why are you calling tonight?" He answered, "I didn't want to ruin your Christmas." Once again, a physician's choices bewildered me. While I appreciated his giving us the results, what timing! What a rationale!

After he hung up the phone, Jim appeared thunderstruck. For him, 'cancer' was a death sentence. I tried to reassure him by reminding him that he had been successfully treated for skin cancers and that the urologist had said his cancer was "very treatable." I doubted what I said made any difference.

Did Jim understand the implication of his cancer being 'stage one'? That he had a relatively low Gleason score, the degree of aggressiveness of a tumor of the prostate, new vocabulary for us. What he heard was that he had cancer. Jim sank into a depression.

Over the years, when Jim had been monosyllabic, I would ask, "Are you OK?" He invariably answered, "I am fine. I am just not my usual ebullient self." Well, if he wasn't always ebullient before and had become frustrated by his memory problems, now there was this.

But, at least, this diagnosis was definitive, and we had to weigh different treatment options ranging from surgery, to seed implants, to 'watch and wait,' to herbal remedies.

Believe it or not, I was grateful for the diagnosis of prostate cancer, because focusing on a treatment plan for the cancer distracted Jim from the problems with his mind. Our internist encouraged us to go to a prostate support group meeting. We did – once. It required talking and was too public for Jim, so I went online. Should we go back north to Memorial Sloan-Kettering Cancer Center in Manhattan?

I had been doing some online editing and had become friends with the operations manager who lived near Boston. I told Belinda about Jim's cancer diagnosis. She immediately contacted an oncologist in Kentucky, who invited us to call him at his home. He also recommended radioactive seed implants and added that the procedure was not 'rocket science.' He said, "There's no need to go to Duke or Sloan-Kettering or to Kentucky to see me; Jim can undergo the treatment just as well in Savannah." We thanked him, and I researched other websites. Jim looked at the printouts, reflected on the phone calls and decided on the method of treatment. His mind was working.

After consultations with the radiation oncologist, the urologist, and the internist, Jim decided to be treated with radioactive seed implants.

The morning of the procedure, I remembered to ask the anesthesiologist to avoid Versed because of Jim's previous paradoxical reaction. He said, "I have never heard of such a thing in adults." I pleaded with him. When Jim came out of the anesthesia, the recovery room nurse asked, "Where are you?" Jim answered, "Paris." She looked at me and asked, "Does he mean it, or is he joking?" I had no idea.

The radioactive seed implants were followed by a short course of external beam radiation. Despite his occasional tears, he was 'of good cheer,' to use his phrase. We walked hand in hand to his appointments. Did he understand the external beam radiation treatments? After each treatment, he said, "They were taking pictures." But afterwards, he cried and said, "My life is useless."

ço ಲ

Jim became sufficiently depressed during the prostate cancer treatment that our internist referred him to a psychiatrist. With Jim's language skills deteriorating, he had difficulty talking with her. She prescribed different antidepressants – none of which worked and most of which resulted in more paradoxical reactions – agitation or greater confusion. The psychiatrist was excited about one particular drug, Remeron, which she thought might alleviate his depression and reduce his tremors – now in his whole hand rather than only in the tip of a finger.

Within half an hour of taking the prescribed dose of Remeron, his lower lip drooped, he began to slur his words, and he was slumped over. He looked 'stoned.' I called the doctor. She said, "Put him to bed and let him sleep it off."

The next morning we had an appointment at a lawyer's office to sign some papers. I spent the evening looking for our durable power of attorney, a document I soon would have to use more than I care to say, including once on a trip to a Social Security Administration Office for me to become Jim's 'representative payee.' By then he had 'sobered up' and was able to sign his name many times – another drug, another reaction.

The psychiatrist also arranged for Jim to have an EEG, an electroencephalogram, which measures brain wave activity. The test required Jim to be sleep-deprived. Because he had to stay up all night, we were both sleep-deprived. The results revealed that Jim's brainwaves were slower than normal. But what did that mean? What were the implications?

ço ಲ

Eventually the radiation treatments exhausted him, and he developed an 'urgency,' which embarrassed him; he didn't want to walk on the beach anymore. He preferred to stay close to the house for fear of wetting himself; he let me help him with some of the nuisances of his treatment. He believed he was dying. He became more withdrawn, and if I asked, "Do you want to go anywhere or do anything today?" his reply was, "What's the point?"

His new blood tests indicated that his PSA was lower, but I told the radiation oncologist that Jim didn't believe that he had been treated successfully. Amazingly, the doctor braved a litigious world and wrote on the back of one of his business cards, "Your cancer is gone," and signed his name. Jim's eyes welled with tears, but he still didn't believe he was cured. The doctor took out a mini-recorder and taped what he had written on the card. Jim put the card in his wallet; the tape went into his top dresser drawer.

ço ✍

During one of our visits, I had mentioned to the urologist my disappointment with the neurologist who had said, "Brain shrinkage." Surely we could find someone with a more definitive diagnosis. So, in the hopes of getting more definitive answers, we arranged to see neurologist number two.

This time, instead of being asked to name presidents, Jim was asked to name as many animals as he could in 60 seconds. Jim named two and sat silent for another 10 or 15 seconds. Then the doctor said, "You have 40 seconds left"; at which point, Jim stood up, reached for my hand and said, "Thank you. We are leaving."

Jim's abrupt desire to leave suggested that he was humiliated or embarrassed by the tests. How would we ever get any information? Our lives were filling with physicians, but we seemed no closer to answers.

៛៛ ៛៛

When the treatment for the prostate cancer was completed, we headed north again. The 800-mile trip was uneventful.

In retrospect, I was the one with the mental deficiency, not Jim. While I could see that life needed to be less stressful for him, it never occurred to me to give up our snowbird lifestyle, that we needed one place, not two.

I did think about our summers, though, and about being closer to the Berkshires, which would be more peaceful for him than the hustle and bustle of New York City.

Having a place in the country, in a part of the world he loved, where he could still enjoy art, music and theatre would be less taxing. There he could see trees and hillsides and walk on a sidewalk at his own pace. I wasn't in denial. His cancer was in check. Why not the cognitive impairment?

While the location was pastoral, I didn't comprehend that his mind and body were being destroyed and how that deterioration would manifest itself. We had been given different labels and drugs to try – mostly for depression – but we had no guidance. I was used to doctors making recommendations the way the urologist had. Here's the problem, here's the treatment: rest in bed, take an aspirin, drink fluids, or take this antibiotic for 10 days. What did 'brain shrinkage' mean? What did 'lapses in memory' mean? What could we do about it? Watch the way he handles the checkbook? Try an antidepressant?

When I suggested moving to the Berkshires, Jim agreed grudgingly.

To make a long story short, in 1999 we bought a condo in Lenox and sold our *pied-à-terre* simultaneously. The market was good then, as was the timing. As I packed, Jim simply sat and watched. In the past, he had scolded me if I lifted something heavy or bulky and would promptly take it out of my hand. The man who packed us in two days to leave Ireland looked bewildered. Everything had fallen into place, except the illness.

Once we moved, I found a part-time job with the folks I had met when I was working with the conference group in the city. I felt a wave of sadness giving up New York City, but we had a gentler world for Jim. I guess I thought Jim would be mildly impaired forever, and my mission was to help him feel less stressed and more secure. I ignored my inner voice that said, "Hey, what about you?" Arrogantly, I thought that if I took care of him, he would be OK. He was just impaired, and, "If you're OK, I'm OK." How naïve!

Not for the first time had I been that arrogant. I had a boss once with a steel-trap mind and a sharp tongue, who used to make us all quake in our shoes. A colleague had said, "She turns us all into gruel." At the time, I told Jim how guilty I felt that my boss's husband had been diagnosed with a brain tumor. "I despise her," I said. "Now look what has happened to her husband." I thought I had wished evil on her. Jim turned to me and shook his head sadly, "Sweetie, don't flatter yourself! There was a long line ahead of you." Now here I was thinking I could make a difference for Jim – 'flattering myself' again.

Once ensconced in Lenox, we went to Tanglewood. At the rehearsals or concerts, Jim sat in his seat with his arms folded, hat pulled down over his face and acknowledged no one. I bought tickets for box seats for some concerts because I wanted Jim to have as much 'special' as we could afford. It was the same reasoning that had prompted me to make a reservation at The Hotel Hershey rather than a Motel 8 or 10 on the trip south. I wanted the best for him. I wanted a chocolate on his pillow.

ॐ ॐ

The truth was we still had no definitive information. Should we see another physician for another opinion? Would someone else have some insight? I thought we should, so we were referred to an osteopath. I explained to him that we had seen several doctors, and I told him about the "brain shrinkage," the "90% sure Alzheimer's," and the "memory lapses." Once again, Jim was asked to perform; I recognized some questions from the previous tests. If he wasn't doing any better on the tests, I was. "Spell 'world' backwards." Jim missed it. But this physician did something different. He put his hands on Jim's arms and wrists and moved them up and down. At the end of his examination, he said, "You don't have Alzheimer's. You have Parkinson's! And it is too early in the illness to use any sort of medication."

"However, for the depression," he added, "I recommend that you see comedies instead of tragedies." So now we had 'memory lapses,' Alzheimer's and Parkinson's, and my thinking about writing a Dummies' book or preparing Cliff Notes on how to pass mini-mental status tests.

Jim didn't react to the diagnosis. I did. Believe it or not, I was elated when I heard Parkinson's. When we got in the car after leaving the osteopath's office, I was giddy. "Sweetie, what great news!" My heart soared. Jim seemed unmoved. I reassured him, "Lots of people have Parkinson's." I rattled off: Hitler, Mohammed Ali, Janet Reno, and Michael J. Fox. "Sure the disease is a bloody nuisance, but it won't kill you." I wasn't in denial. Once again, I didn't understand the implications, and I hadn't asked what they were.

ఞ ఞ

A few days later, I woke up with a sharp pain in my side. *No!* I guessed what was wrong. Before heading north for the summer, my gynecologist had admonished me, "Your fibroid is so big, I am concerned that it is going to damage your kidney. You should have a hysterectomy." I had said, "Jim's not well. I can't deal with this now. How about when we get back in the fall?" So I had a good idea what was causing the pain. Increasingly leery of physicians, I saw a local gynecologist who recommended surgery. He said, "The fibroid isn't the biggest I've ever seen." Once again I was dismayed by a physician's communication skills. Was fibroid size a competition? In any event, the fibroid was pushing on my kidney; I needed a hysterectomy. Apparently it was surgery or kidney damage.

Once again I called Belinda, who found a physician in Cambridge. We went. He examined me. We talked. I argued against having the surgery; he parried my arguments. I was worried because I was concerned about Jim, and I knew I would be unable to drive or lift anything; I also was disappointed about giving up my part-time job. Meanwhile, I was aware that Jim was changing.

Regardless, we scheduled the surgery. Jim actually said to me, "Get it over with." I booked a hotel room near the hospital and arranged for a limo for the roundtrip. A day before the surgery, we went to a Van Gogh exhibit at the Museum of Fine Arts. The morning of the surgery, Belinda and her daughter, Catrina, met us and chauffeured Jim to and from the hospital and made sure he ate. While he knew how to find his hotel room once inside the hotel, he could not take taxis or buses or get meals at restaurants on his own.

Did he understand I was having surgery? I wasn't sure. The morning of the surgery, he held my hand. But when I was discharged a couple of days later, barely able to walk or stand up straight, my darling husband said, "I'm bored." I promised to go to the Fogg Museum, if he would wait until the next morning. The museum was a five-minute walk from the hotel – if you are healthy. I managed to walk at a snail's pace and climb up the steps. While Jim admired the art, I sat on a bench in the rotunda holding my belly, hoping that whatever was left inside wouldn't fall out. Was he aware of my discomfort? My normally loving, attentive husband no longer seemed concerned for me.

Before leaving for Boston, I had stocked our freezer full of frozen dinners, so once we were back home, all I had to do was walk from the freezer to the microwave; Jim no longer cooked. I tried to walk as much as possible and to be a role-model for 'recovery.' When we returned to Boston for a follow-up visit, the gynecologist said, "The pathology report indicated that you had stage one endometrial cancer. You are very lucky, and you have been treated." In essence, it was a good thing that I had the surgery when I did, and I was determined to show Jim that cancer was nothing. Did he understand? His own illness was depressing him. Was it the prostate cancer? Was he confused because he was depressed? Was he depressed because he was confused? We went to see another psychiatrist.

❧ ❧

Jim called this doctor, "the Professor", and he trusted him and saw him once a week throughout the summer. We walked to his office, where I would leave him while they talked "haltingly." Once again, the Professor, like the other physicians, tried different medications to lift Jim's spirits – Wellbutrin and Dexadrine were two. I already had a shoebox filled with bottles of pills and samples. Nothing worked. Jim's reactions were dramatic and/or paradoxical.

Around then, we had lunch with a friend from my commuting days and a friend of his who was a psychiatric social worker. After the meal, she took Jim aside and suggested that he go to New York for another diagnosis – and then added that he deserved to be happier. My diffident Jim kissed her on the cheek and said, "Thank you."

We all hoped that depression was affecting his memory. With the Professor's blessing, we made an appointment to see a psychiatrist in New York City. By then we had seen two neurologists, one internist, two psychiatrists, an osteopath and a psychologist, and we still didn't have an answer.

৩ ৯

We had just had our annual eye exams. Because Jim had never cared for his progressive lenses, the change in his prescription was an opportunity for him to get separate glasses: one for reading, one for distance and a third pair of distance sunglasses. Each pair had a different frame. When we got home from the optician, Jim put all three pairs on the bed and tried and tried to figure out which glasses were for what purpose. For close to an hour, I tried to explain that the frames were different on each of the different glasses and what each pair of glasses was for. Why couldn't he understand? He got angry and frustrated. So did I.

As a consequence, we returned to the optician the next day and ordered new glasses – a single pair of photosensitive, Varilux lenses – one pair of glasses for everything. Change was hard for him – any change.

৩ ৯

Armed with his new glasses, we went into the city to see the new psychiatrist. She added new words to our expanding vocabulary. Her diagnosis: dysthymia, chronic depression and some neurological problem; her phrase was "neurological substrate." She didn't say, "Parkinson's." She didn't say, "Alzheimer's." She didn't ask Jim to count backwards; instead, she asked him to write out "Mary had a little lamb" on a pad. As he wrote, I saw how his once beautiful, open handwriting was now tiny – what's the Parkinson's word? – 'crabbed.' How had I not noticed? How rarely he put pen to paper anymore. She wrote a prescription for Prozac, another antidepressant.

Alzheimer's? Parkinson's disease? Cognitive impairment? Depression? Chronic depression? A neurological substrate? What happened to physicians' examining you and saying, "You have the flu, or chicken pox, or a kidney stone?" What did any of this mean? Was there anything we could do?

With an ever-widening vocabulary and more drugs to avoid, we returned south. Jim had visibly deteriorated by the time he saw his radiation oncologist for a follow-up visit. Drawn and thinner, Jim smiled that endearing smile of his when he entered the physician's office, saw the office staff and the doctor, but his comprehension and language skills had declined, and he was processing information even more slowly. His answers to questions were more labored, and Jim seemed bewildered by being in the examining room. The doctor repeated what he had said at our previous visit, "Your cancer is gone." Jim sobbed. Then the oncologist asked, "Jim, are you having any discomfort?" Jim did not respond. The doctor took me aside and asked, "Do you think he understood what I asked him?" Then privately he said, "I am concerned by the rapid changes in Jim's mental and physical condition."

We stopped checking his PSA. How would he have reacted to his having a needle stuck in his arm? And to what end?

ഏ ൙

Frustrated by the lack of information and medical response in the South, I had asked my gynecologist in Cambridge for a referral to a neurologist at a teaching hospital in Boston, but when I phoned for an appointment, I was told we would have to wait months. With winter coming, I asked our internist in the South if he could refer us to a neurologist at a teaching hospital. The first available appointment was at the end of November.

Jim was so nervous about being late to that appointment that he awoke at 4:00 am. The drive was two hours, the appointment at 10:00 am. When we arrived, the neurologist walked out of his office, stood in the hallway, smiled, extended his hand and welcomed us as we walked down the corridor. He invited us into his office, offered us chairs and asked Jim, "How was the drive?" Jim was looking out the window at the bridges and rooftops of Charleston. "How do you like the view? How was your summer?" Jim answered each question slowly, but he answered. Then the neurologist asked Jim's permission to check his reflexes. Jim was relaxed. He chatted. He smiled. He didn't stand up and leave. While he groped for words, he seemed neither frightened nor intimidated, and Jim was not asked to perform. The doctor seemed to evaluate him, without mini-mental status tests. Apparently, the walk down the corridor, the handshake, the conversation and the examination of his reflexes enabled the neurologist to determine what was happening, while maintaining Jim's dignity. On the ride back, Jim referred to the neurologist as a "gentleman." In his notes, the neurologist referred to Jim as a "gentleman" as well.

Jim saw the neurologist several times. At first, he diagnosed Jim with "cognitive decline" and "parkinsonism," a condition that causes a combination of movement abnormalities – no other label. I had explained about the paradoxical reaction to Versed and Jim's drug sensitivity in general. Still no definitive diagnosis and no symptomatic relief from drugs, but we had a neurologist who smiled and treated Jim with more dignity.

૭ ન૭

After one of our appointments with the neurologist, I asked if I might speak to him alone. I asked him, "What is happening to Jim?" I asked for a diagnosis and a prognosis. His answer? "You got a bad hand." The prognosis? Jim would become more tired over time.

For more definitive information, he suggested that we see a particular neuropsychiatrist. We did, and once again, Jim had to undergo psychological tests, while I waited in another room until they finished. After the testing was completed, the physician took me into another room and spoke to me privately.

The afternoon had begun with, "How can we help you?" It ended with the physician telling me that Jim might have Gertsmann's Syndrome, or Lewy Body Disease, or something else with a Latin, Greek or German name. Not knowing what those labels meant, I repeated what I had asked before, "What do I do?" He said: "Don't buy a boat or a 10,000 square foot house." This physician said, "Don't buy a boat or a 10,000 square foot house"! The love of my life didn't know who he was, or who I was, and the medical advice was: "Don't buy a boat"? *Somebody help us, please! Oh, please!*

What's the tally? Two for Alzheimer's, two for cognitive impairment, one for Parkinson's, one for Parkinsonism, one for Gertsmann's, maybe, or Lewy Body Dementia, and don't forget dysthymia with a neurological substrate.

On the drive back, Jim looked at me. He said, "What's wrong with me? Do I have cancer of the brain? Do I need to be put away?" His questions were heartrending. I could only reassure him that he didn't have 'cancer of the brain,' and "No, he didn't need to be put away." But how could I help that dear, sweet man? What was wrong? For sure, I knew we weren't going to buy a boat.

ళ అ

Amazingly or idiotically, we returned to Lenox for the following summer. Jim resumed seeing the Professor, who suggested we go to the Memory Disorders Program at the Berkshire Medical Center. There we met a charming woman, who offered practical suggestions like labeling objects and putting glasses and keys in the same place. She also referred us to another neurologist, our fourth, who, like the neurologist in the teaching hospital, was gracious and smiling and did not put Jim through his paces with quizzes and tests. Jim was at ease with her.

After examining him, she diagnosed him with Lewy Body Dementia (LBD), a disease that is difficult to diagnose; it is similar to Alzheimer's and to Parkinson's. Researchers were only beginning to study those similarities and differences, but in LBD, there is mental decline, sleep disturbances, hallucinations, depression and early psychoses.

In the fall, a fifth neurologist in Charleston corroborated her diagnosis. He too said Jim was suffering from Lewy Body Dementia. He recommended that I go online and look at www.lewynet.com. One of the hallmarks of the illness is drug sensitivity. Only an autopsy would have told us for sure.

ᘧ ᘨ

That final summer of 2001 in Lenox was tragic. While we had made the drive north, it was only a matter of weeks after our arrival before Jim became profoundly confused. He didn't know he had a right to be in his own apartment, and occasionally he didn't know me. On some days he let me know I frightened him. Other days, he put his wallet, razor and glasses in a plastic bag and carried them with him all day. He was becoming 'paranoid.'

Another day, we drove to a dermatologist. During the entire trip, Jim kept turning around to look in the back seat for the person he believed was sitting there and who was not. He was 'hallucinating.'

He continued going to his appointments with the Professor, but he rarely spoke anymore. When the Professor asked him where he lived, Jim said, "Yonkers." His body was suffering, too. He seemed more rigid and his tremor more pronounced.

Because of his increasing stiffness, I encouraged him to come with me to a gym to walk on a treadmill. He did a few times. I even tried to have him work with a personal trainer and to try some yoga. But he could not follow directions, so that was that.

One evening, before going to Tanglewood – which we still did – he asked me, "How will the ushers know which seats are ours? How will the ushers know our seats?" He repeated the questions over and over again. I didn't know how to talk to a confused man. He was anxious, and we had the 'conversation' for over half an hour.

Once again I bought box seats for the final concert of the season, Beethoven's *Ninth*. I finally grasped the fact that our lives were changing irrevocably. What I knew for sure was that we weren't coming back North. I fought back tears, as I listened to the Boston Symphony and looked at Jim beside me.

I also realized that I could not make the drive back south alone with Jim in his current condition. I needed help. He was too agitated. I asked friends, but the timing wasn't convenient. Then my neighbor offered, but she needed to wait for a few weeks, and we were already seeing snow flurries, so I called a friend in Boston. I asked, "If I fly you back, would you drive south with us?" Maggie said, "Yes."

We picked the day, packed and began the drive. For the first five hours, Jim was his old self, and I was feeling foolish about needing someone to come with us. We stopped for coffee along the New York State Thruway. Jim and Maggie actually chatted about politics – slowly, but they chatted. We climbed back in the car and drove on to Allentown where we stopped for lunch, but this time, when he got back in the car, he became fearful. "Where are we going? Call the police. Turn around. We are driving the wrong way." He was panicked. He calmed down when Maggie reached between the seats and took hold of his hand.

I didn't know what to do. *Should I turn around? Should I go forward?* I gripped the wheel. I tried to talk to him rationally. I continued driving. *North or South? Lenox or Hilton Head? Small apartment or bigger apartment? Snow or sun?* I decided to drive to the sun, the warmth and the additional space. *Do I drive all night? Can I drive straight through? What will he do, if we stop?* I was scared.

The closer we got to Washington DC, the more agitated he became. He was waiting for "orders." I wondered why. Could it have been because I had turned on the TV on September 11, and he had watched the towers collapse? That morning he had sat glued to the set with tears rolling down his cheeks. What had he understood? Now he seemed paranoid. Were the images still in his head? He used words like "power" and "control." I couldn't understand. He spoke of "them." I had no idea who "them" was. Maggie kept holding his hand.

We needed to stop, so we found a Cracker Barrel. What would he do? He got out of the car as calmly as you please. He went to the men's room on his own. We got a bite to eat. He was fine. Then we got back in the car to leave, and he stared at me and said, "You stole my money! What did you do with my money?"

Again Maggie held his hand and assured him that he was OK. At this point he made an introduction. He looked at me and said, "This is my wife." He was introducing Maggie, as his wife, to me.

Maggie held his hand for the next several hundred miles. With my heart in my throat, we stopped for the night; once again, he climbed out of the car as if everything was fine. We went to the restaurant; he ordered a hamburger, and after dinner, we went to our rooms. I was afraid to be alone with him. Maggie was in the adjoining room and told me to phone her if I needed help. Jim climbed into bed in the strange room and fell asleep; I climbed into bed and stayed awake.

The next morning I was tired and ached from the tension. I drove to Hilton Head and parked outside our condo. Jim opened the car door, got out, went right upstairs to our apartment, took the key, unlocked the door, walked in and headed for the bathroom. He knew where he was. I, on the other hand, was exhausted. We never went north together again.

ৎ৵ ৵৹

Now paranoid and delusional, Jim was also having spatial problems. He seemed to have difficulty differentiating between a hole, a dark space or a shadow on the floor; he urinated in the wastebasket rather than the toilet. He was increasingly and more frequently 'paranoid.' Believing people were stealing from him, he hid his wallet, his glasses and his Ferragamo loafers. Later in his illness, he would still hide them, but in plain sight – on the floor at the foot of the bed.

By now we had another new internist. As compassionate and helpful as our previous one had been, Jim could not, and would not, sit in a waiting room for an hour and a half to see him. The new internist met Jim and recommended that we try Paxil for his anxiety. Once again, the Paxil made him more anxious and more paranoid. I assumed and hoped, like the doctors, that perhaps some small amount of some medication might help him, but one part of a tablet invariably told the whole story.

Because the Parkinsonism caused him problems with his movement and rigidity, I asked the internist for a referral for Jim to have some physical therapy, hoping that it might help, even though going to the gym had been a bust. Thankfully, the doctor did and also referred him for occupational therapy as well. That failed, but his meeting with the physical therapist was a resounding success.

His physical therapist, Denny, was a retired marine, and they hit it off instantly. We went to the Rehab Center three times a week. Denny gave Jim some simple exercises like walking on the treadmill or riding on a stationary bike for a few minutes. Denny was friendly, patient and persistent, and Jim was completely at ease. They also walked on uneven ground together to help him maintain his balance. Happily, I wrote a story for a Savannah paper about Denny's remarkable career change.

৩ ৫

During the visit in which the new internist had written the prescription for Paxil and for rehab, with Jim within earshot, it was suggested that it was over and that I should put him away.

It's over? Put him away? I still hear those words. Whatever "IT" was, "IT" wasn't over. I adored this man. *Over! For better or for worse, … in sickness and in health.* This man being talked about and apparently dismissed was my husband. "Put him away"? Well, that was another matter altogether, one that I hadn't thought about, and Jim had asked several times, "Do I need a home?"

That night and the next and the next, I thought about what had been said. *Was that something I should consider? Would Jim be better off in a facility? Would he get better care than I could give him at home? Would a nursing home be a safer environment for him? Would he be happier?*

I was familiar with facilities like that. My dad had lived in a nursing home for years. My grandmother had lived in a retirement home, too, and I knew people with family in nursing homes. I dismissed with contempt the first part of the statement about it's being over. But I said to myself, maybe, maybe I should try 'putting him away.'

The opportunity arose to try a facility when Jim went through another bad patch; he was so confused I had taken him to the local hospital again, thinking naïvely that trained medical professionals might help him better than I could. He was admitted. I could have stayed overnight with him, but I didn't know I had that option. Once he was settled in his room, I left him alone and went home. What was I thinking!

When I returned at 6:30 in the morning, a nurse said, "Mr. Tierney got out of bed and was walking around the corridors looking for his wife." "Why didn't you call me?" I asked. They had no answer to that. The solution? They gave him Ativan for sleep. And they gave this confused, drug-sensitive, ambulatory dementia patient more than one dose. When I arrived, he was in bed – out cold. When he finally came out of his drugged state, he could barely sit up, much less stand, and, when he did, he managed to climb out of bed, moving like a drunk and promptly urinated on the floor.

This was the morning that the social workers from the different nursing homes and assisted-living facilities were scheduled to evaluate him. When they came into his room, what they saw was a helpless man who could barely stand; the assisted-living residences rejected him. In fact, only one skilled nursing home accepted him.

Because he was being discharged from a hospital directly to a nursing home, Medicare paid the charges. A courtesy van took us to the facility. Everyone was gracious. I was feeling hopeful. Maybe a 'home' would be better for him. The administration understood we were 'trying it out' for two weeks.

Jim was given a pretty room with a couch for me. I slept when Jim did, woke up quietly around 3:00 am, tiptoed out to go home, shower, change and return by 4:00. I selected his meals from a list of splendid choices. We were served at a long table in a private dining room where other patients ate as well – unaided. Jim only said, "Hello."

But why did they wake him by turning on his lights at midnight to check on him? Why were breakfast, shift change and shower all scheduled for 7:00? The staff could only do so much, so I helped him shower, dress and go to the breakfast room by 7:00. I thought, "What is going to happen if I am not here to help?" Meanwhile, Jim kept saying, "I want to go back over the bridge." True, I understood that he needed time to adjust, but what was I doing? How long could I keep driving back and forth in the middle of the night to be sure that he was showered, dressed and ready for breakfast? And, no surprise, the staff readily accepted my help.

For Jim to remain Medicare-eligible at the facility, he needed physical therapy, and he refused it. Quite simply, he would not participate, unless the "leader," Denny, approved. Denny did not work at the nursing facility; he worked at the Rehab Center. Jim was adamant; the leader had to approve. Clearly, he wasn't going to meet Medicare's requirements.

During the week, a minister came into Jim's room, sat down on the sofa beside him and patted his hand. "You are a Catholic, aren't you?" he said. Jim looked down at the hand resting on his own, lifted the man's hand and removed it, then graciously said, "Excuse me, my wife and I are late to lunch." Jim took my hand and walked me out of the room with the bewildered minister looking on.

Jim didn't meet Medicare's requirements at the time; he wanted to go home, and I was pooped. I had gone home as usual in the middle of the night, but this time, I had delayed my return until mid-afternoon. When I returned, Jim was packing and wanted to go back "over the bridge." We went home. I had tried 'putting him away' – for all of a week.

After our sojourn I was more determined to maintain Jim at home, to give him care and security and whatever modicum of joy I could. Being at home meant no schedules and no other residents. He could wake up when he wanted, take an hour to eat, or start a meal and finish it later. He could eat what I knew he liked – fish, seafood and more fish. He could shower when he was ready – once a day or twice – and have one-on-one care.

ক্ল ঞ্চ

But I was pragmatic enough to understand that, if I became seriously ill or died, Jim would need care, so a nursing home still might be in his future. Periodically over the years, I visited different facilities. All but one experience left me feeling uncomfortable.

In one instance I made an appointment, and the interviewer failed to keep it, phone to cancel or reschedule. One Sunday, I deliberately dropped in on another expensive nursing home and waited patiently while two women behind the reception desk sorted out their personal business. Finally, one looked over at me and said, "What do YOU want?" I asked, "Would you show me around?" The two women debated with each other about which one of them would take me on my tour. Once they decided, and we began to walk around, I saw people in their wheelchairs in corners, aides talking to each other over the heads of the residents as they fed them; the subject matter was not the patient. I thought that if they were this ungracious to me – cognitively unimpaired – how would they treat someone helpless and dependent, like Jim. I thanked them for the tour and their time.

Jim and I drove together to another facility that specialized in memory care. I had called ahead. When we got out of the car, the marketing director raced out to meet us, put her arm around Jim, pressed her hip to his and walked him around the building. We looked at the fireplace, the flowers, the glazed eyes watching the TV, the card players, and thanked everyone and left.

What Jim remembered often surprised me: when we went back another time, he climbed back in the car as soon as he saw the same marketing director.

From time to time, I visited different facilities. The quality changed constantly. If the state cited them, they improved. Or if a head of nursing resigned, a facility might deteriorate.

I revisited the nursing home in which my mother died. This time the corridors smelled of urine – not what I expected from previous visits.

I realized I had to stay healthy. Determined to find a place, I visited the facilities in the area, and one day I found a small, loving nursing home and felt secure that it would stay that way and be perfect for Jim should something happen to me.

Nursing homes are institutions. They have to feed, bathe and care for their residents on schedules. No federal law governs the ratio for care, but one aide to eight patients was typical. The given is that patients need constant and differing care, and problems and emergencies happen.

I began to hear stories about nursing homes: the one about the Parkinson's patient with the severe tremor whose food tray was put in front of him; unable to feed himself, he lost 15 pounds in two weeks. Or the one about the frail patient who died from a concussion after two aides dropped her, while transferring her from the chair to the bed. I heard about bedsores out of control, fraud, theft, broken bones unnoticed and dehydration. In essence, someone has to be there to check. Would Jim have been able to use a call bell?

∽ ∾

Although our internist had referred us to Rehab, and the suggestion about a nursing home might have been well-intentioned, I was still reeling from, "It's over. Put him away." I was not writing Jim off. I was writing this physician off. But rather than leave immediately, I decided to shop for a compassionate internist with good communication skills, who believed that Jim deserved to be treated with dignity in an office that wouldn't require us to sit for a long time – something Jim could no longer do.

Because my search was slow, we saw our current internist again at the hospital. Jim had some rectal bleeding again, and I had taken him to the Emergency Room; once again, he was admitted. This time, it was simply bleeding hemorrhoids, but I said I was staying overnight in his room. The next morning when our internist made the rounds, Jim grinned and said, "Good to see you again." The doctor smiled back, thanked him and, walking out of the room with me, said with amazement, "He's still there!" "Yes," I said, "he's still there." I refrained from saying what I wanted to say, which was, "It's not over!"

≫ ≪

To find a more empathetic physician to meet my needs and Jim's, I asked for referrals from nurses, doctors, dentists, and pharmacists. Our internist seemed to have made a decision about Jim, and, therefore, as far as I was concerned, about me as well. After all the doctors we had seen, all the drugs we had tried that had caused problems, I was no longer looking for cures or treatments for Jim's condition. And, if indeed he was suffering from Lewy Body Dementia, there were no cures, no treatments, but at least we had a caring neurologist in Charleston to phone. Painful as it was, I accepted that nothing could be done. The disease had him in its clutches. What I could do was keep him comfortable, safe and well-fed. I could keep him as healthy as possible, while his body and mind were being destroyed. But should something dramatic happen, should he fall and hurt himself or break a bone, or develop some other sorts of symptoms, I wanted someone local to turn to, and I wanted to have the same doctor for myself. To understand me was to understand that Jim was part of my life. I began my search.

I was referred to an osteopath. I explained that I was looking for a physician for myself and, if need be, for my husband. I described Jim's condition. He said, "In Canada, when people can't feed themselves, they are allowed to die. You aren't giving him a flu shot, are you? You aren't giving him vitamins, are you?" I said "No" to the flu shot question and avoided answering the one about the vitamins.

I left his office and got into my car. Not only was the disease a "bad hand," I also felt as if we had no one on our side except our neurologist two hours away. Did medical folks believe you stop loving or wanting to help someone because they have a dementing illness? Jim was still there with blinding and, at times, hilarious glimpses of the man he used to be.

I phoned the doctor of Integrative Medicine we had seen in New York. We had met her when we were living near the city; at the time, I still hoped that nutritional changes might help him. Vitamin B? Vitamin D? So, here I was, sitting in my car in Hilton Head, feeling lonelier and lonelier. I was losing Jim, and I felt alone without support. No, I was not giving him a flu shot, but, yes, I was giving Jim vitamins and protein powder – for his skin – to keep him healthy and help protect against pressure sores.

The doctor returned my call within minutes. I told her what the osteopath had just said to me. She was angry, "It is NOT your job to be the grim reaper! Jim will die in his time. If it makes you feel better to give him vitamins to make him more comfortable, then do it." My tears were no longer from frustration; they were because of her kindness. Why did it seem so hard for so many other members of the medical community to understand that I wanted the best for my husband, regardless of his condition? She did.

I was referred to yet another osteopath. Once again, I told him about Jim's condition and explained that I was shopping, but this time I blurted out, "I need to know if your compassion was removed when you went to medical school?" Unphased by my bitter remark, he said, "Jim is preparing to meet God." I listened and thanked him for his time.

I met another internist who quoted Scripture. I said, "Please, I am not a religious person." He said, 'It doesn't matter. I am." He continued his recitation from *The Bible*. I thanked him as well.

These physicians made our neurologist unforgettable by comparison. He had treated Jim as the man he used to be and me with respect. He was sensitive to the tragedy. He was kind. He returned my phone calls. If Jim was constipated, which he was; if his legs wouldn't support him, which they didn't; if he suddenly walked tilted to one side, which he did, the neurologist would take the time to make a suggestion, knowing that what he was saying might or might not work.

During my search, I was reminded of our doctor's words in Chatham in the 1980s when he had decided to give up his private practice to go into research. We liked him and were concerned about having to find another physician of his caliber. He said, "Don't worry. The medical schools are turning out great technicians." They were technicians, yes, but not always empathetic communicators.

Eventually I found wonderful physicians, but it took time. One was our dermatologist. Jim had fair Irish skin and frequently had been treated for precancerous and cancerous lesions. The dermatologist scolded me for bringing an agitated and confused Jim to the office. "I can go to your home. I live nearby. Next time, call and say that you need me to come by." I couldn't believe it. I called, and he came – many times. We met an optician who offered to make a house call to adjust Jim's glasses. He did. Our dentist came to the house to check Jim's teeth when we found he had lost a crown.

Eventually I was referred to an internist who took care of my health. She honored my decision to keep Jim at home and offered to help in any way she could. Rather than advising me to 'put him away', she applauded my strength for keeping him at home.

Pharmacists became allies, too. For example, when Jim had relentless hiccups, one pharmacist suggested shifting his position. Whatever his latest symptom, I could ask for advice and they gave it. I walked into the store one day and broke down. The pharmacist said, "You have made it this far. You can do it." What a difference it made when someone said, "Hang in there," rather than "What's the matter with you? Put him in a nursing home and get on with your life."

PART THREE

There's a kind of release and a kind of torment in every
goodbye for every man.

C. Day-Lewis

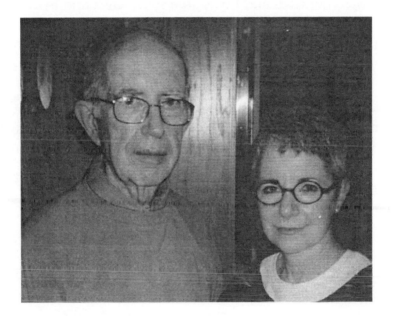

Four years after Jim's initial diagnosis, I was exhausted. Nothing in our lives was normal anymore. If I ran an errand by myself or went to a yoga class, I would have one eye on my watch, or would roll up my mat halfway into the practice. If I did stay through a class, I would be asking myself how this illness had happened to us and desperately wanting my old Jim back. When I left him alone at home, I was always in a hurry, fearful that he might become agitated or confused; I wasn't concerned about his hurting himself or wandering off.

Several times I had returned home to find him holding his head saying, "I'm going to my funeral," or staring out the window looking for a car, for his car or for a red car. Because he had difficulty concentrating, he no longer wanted or needed time 'to read.' Hoping it might help, I bought CDs of poetry, and I ordered a tape player and audio books for the blind. Not only was he not interested, he was unable to push the oversized buttons on the machine; he had nothing to keep him occupied.

He was confused, and I was on a short leash and irritable. A telemarketing call at the wrong time, a brief wait at a checkout counter, a letter addressed to someone else – everything annoyed me out of proportion to the event.

It was easier to run errands together, but that was problematic, too. If we drove to the bank or to the store, he reprimanded me for driving in the wrong direction, just as he had on our final trip south. He tried to open the door of the car when it was in motion, or to unbuckle his seatbelt when I came to a stop sign or red light. I was on guard and on edge.

Inside a store, his behavior was equally unpredictable; while I was at the checkout counter, credit card in one hand, emptying the cart as fast as I could with the other, he might bolt for the door. When I was at a teller's window or at the post office counter, he would demand to see the manager. I completed my transactions as fast as possible to catch up with him, steer him back to the car or simply walk after him.

At home, he followed me everywhere. If I talked on the phone, he talked to me simultaneously. If I needed a few quiet minutes to sit, or write or complete paperwork, there were none. I couldn't concentrate. The checkbook was unbalanced. My last entry on my Quicken software was months earlier. I mailed letters without stamps, put the wrong checks in envelopes, paid the wrong amounts, wrote checks, put them in stamped envelopes and forgot to mail them, so I was assessed late charges. I sorted through a pile of papers and found unmailed letters and a two-year old check I had failed to deposit. Jim's behavior was 'quixotic,' and I was in a state. Because I couldn't stay on hold with a customer service representative at Blue Shield or Medicare, I found a woman who ran a small business helping people file insurance claims. I registered with her, and she handled that chore for us.

Poor Jim was so confused. One quiet afternoon, we drove to the local Barnes & Noble because it offered a familiar layout and also was a place to walk, no longer a place to buy. We strolled around the store, and when we were done, I asked if he wanted to go to Pier One, which was next door. He said, "You mean in Dalton?" Dalton? Barnes & Noble was next door to Pier One in Dalton, just north of Lenox. We were in Hilton Head at the time.

ॐ ॐ

Besides the bookstore, another familiar place to go was the local deli. We had eaten lox and cream cheese on rye there for years. On one particular visit, Herman, the owner, joined us and regaled us with stories about the old days in the Bronx. Jim listened, seemed to understand and laughed. Then Herman finished his sandwich and got up from the table. We finished ours. I paid, and we walked to the car. I opened the passenger's door for Jim; he climbed in, and I walked around and got in the driver's side and helped him with his seatbelt. As I buckled him in, he looked at me and smiled. "That was fun," he said. Then he paused, continued staring at me and asked, "But who are you?"

My heart sank. His not recognizing me was happening more and more frequently; he would look frightened, or stare at me and then dart away. And my saying, "I am Elizabeth, your wife," was a waste of time! I was sick at heart and personalizing his rejection.

How could he not recognize me? Not only did he not know me, I had become a group of strangers – some disturbing, others benign. The 'driver' of the car – me – was one person. The person in the kitchen another, and the one in the front room of the apartment, the one with the computer, seemed to be the "manager" or "supervisor" – the least amiable of the bunch. When we were standing in the living room, he would look toward that room, lower his voice and ask me, "Where is SHE?"

Shortly thereafter, we were going to take a walk. We left our apartment and proceeded along the walkway down the stairs to the second floor. But, instead of going down the stairs to the first floor, Jim suddenly turned back along the walkway to the apartment door directly below ours. We lived on the third floor. We were standing on the second floor in front of the apartment door that looked exactly like ours, except it was #202 not #302. Jim turned the knob of that door. It wouldn't open. And no one was home. I told him that he was turning the knob of the wrong door, but he continued to turn it, and the more he tried, the more frustrated he got. I stood beside him. I walked away. I came back. I watched. I explained that our apartment was one flight up. He didn't listen to me. Eventually, I walked down the stairs to the first floor and yelled up, "Jim, come on down. That's not our apartment." He wouldn't budge. He continued trying to open the door of the second floor apartment door, which would not open. I walked back up to the third floor and shouted down to him. Then I walked down the stairs to the first floor again. What should I do? What could I do?

I was stunned watching my adored husband. What had happened to him and to me? Once again, I told him that he was at the wrong apartment. He yelled at me, "Get up here, Frank."

Our condo was in a gated community, so, in desperation and with a sense of humiliation, I used my cell phone to call Security and explained what was happening. A guard drove over. I couldn't hear what he said, but he spoke softly to Jim, who smiled at him and walked without hesitation back up to the third floor. "Frank" lacked that touch.

ஒ ஒ

To date, my education about dementia consisted of what I had been taught at the Memory Disorders Program, from the doctors whose advice ranged from not buying a boat, going to comedies instead of tragedies or saying that Jim would become more tired. I remained uneducated about the disease and its progression.

I remembered a book that a social worker had suggested years earlier for my mother to read. At the time, I had only skimmed it. I bought another copy of the classic, *The 36 Hour Day*.

In search of answers, I found and went to several meetings of the local chapter of an Alzheimer's support group, but more often than not, I was the only person at the session run by a social worker with an, 'Oh, dear, I am so sorry' voice. I wanted to say, "Instead of feeling sorry for me, help me. Make him better. Help me help him. Tell me what to do. Make him remember me. I can't bear this, and I can't believe it. Help. I don't know what to do." I didn't. I saved my rants for elsewhere – in the shower, in the car, on the street – anytime. However, at the support group, I learned the word, 'respite.' I stopped going to the meetings because it was too stressful to leave Jim alone in order to have someone tell me I needed a 'break.'

ஒ ஒ

I tried to learn what to do by watching him. For example, we had two large built-in mirrors in the apartment: one was along a section of wall, the other a wall-to-floor mirror behind the bathtub. I had noticed Jim seemed upset by the reflections at sunset, or by the light when he walked by those mirrors. What was he seeing? How did he interpret what he was seeing? Did he recognize himself? Was it someone else? I covered both mirrors, one with a drape and the other with a shower curtain. It seemed to help.

I stopped watching television on the day he yelled, "Fire!" He had been in the bedroom, and the flickering lights reflected on the wall in the living room must have frightened him.

I also had noticed that, when Jim walked around the apartment or outside, from time to time he raised his foot to take a bigger step, as if to avoid something in his path. I paid more attention. The bigger step seemed to occur when there was a shadow, or a different texture or color on the ground or floor. At home I tried full spectrum light bulbs, hoping that they would make a difference. I couldn't do much about shadows of clouds or trees on the grass; however, I removed the patterned bathroom mats and replaced them with a big, slip-proof, solid-colored mat that matched the color of the bathroom floor and the carpet. It seemed to help. While I worried about the possibility of his slipping, with incontinence, 'washable' also mattered.

I also stopped speaking so quickly with him and learned to wait for him to process what I was saying. I would say or ask something slowly, then wait and watch his face for an answer or a reaction – no more quick decisions or brilliant repartee.

While Jim didn't always know my face, he always recognized voices on the telephone. I would hold the receiver to his ear; he would hear the voice and say the correct name. A friend of mine had been diagnosed with Alzheimer's; her husband noticed that she, too, recognized voices on the phone.

So, when Jim was particularly upset because he had no car, no home or no money, I would phone one of his children or our accountant and put Jim on the line, hoping that a familiar voice might ground him. By the end of the call, he was usually calmer.

His son, Kevin, called him once a week without fail. Jim immediately recognized the voice and said, "Kevin," and then chatted away – often unintelligibly. One time after finishing the call, and I had hung up the phone for him, Jim said "Good man"; another time, he said, "Good-bye, Son."

Kevin visited once a year. The first year, when Kevin walked in, Jim's smile lit up the room. We all went out to lunch and then for ice cream. The next year, when Kevin came, we tried the same thing, but Jim would not get out of the car. The following year, there were no more car rides. Instead, Kevin helped the aides and sat by his father's recliner and held his hand, while Jim muttered in a language largely unfamiliar to us all.

ço ∾

Jim's behavior was becoming more aberrant and for longer periods of time, and I didn't know what to do. No longer good days and bad, it was good hours and bad ones, good minutes and bad ones. He was normal or abnormal, calm or agitated.

He said, "I have no money." He said, "I have no home." Someone was being "murdered." He ripped the bedding. He moved the furniture. He hid his glasses, wallet, belt, shoes under the bed, in his dresser drawers, in the closet or in his pockets. People were stealing from him – including me. Apparently, strange people surrounded him. He threatened me when I didn't return the "stones." His clothes weren't his. "I can't wear these," he said, "they belong to O'Neill." He needed help; he no longer knew how to use the shower. He frequently shouted for the police. He was leaving home – to go home. One night he got up and packed a shopping bag with a pair of shoes, some incontinence underwear and a belt and headed for the door to "catch a plane."

One morning he broke my heart yet again, when he ceremoniously handed me his precious Ferragamo loafers and said, "Thank you."

ॐ ঐ

Nor was Jim sleeping at night. Just as he had the night he packed his shopping bag, he would awaken in the middle of the night, get out of bed, walk around – sometimes with no clothes on – and turn the lights on and off or stand at a light switch flicking it on and off for 10 or 15 minutes. The darkness and dim lighting may have made me seem more frightening because on several nights he chased me around the apartment demanding the return of the "stones." He often demanded the return of the "stones." I never knew what they were, but he wanted them back.

One particular night when he chased me, I ran into the front room, locked the door and clutched the phone to my chest. I was afraid of my own husband, of my once gentle Jim. How could this be happening? About a half an hour later, I cracked open the door, peeked out and tiptoed back toward our bedroom. I stood back from the bedroom door, ready to run again. I watched Jim while he moved the furniture and stripped the bed. Eventually, he lay down halfway across the unmade bed and fell asleep.

One morning, he warned me about the Jews – this from my Yeshiva teacher and Rogers Peet "goy." What were the Jews doing? I couldn't make it out, but something bad – this random utterance from one of the most humanistic, ecumenical people I ever met. What Jim said he didn't tolerate was "stupidity and Irish politicians!" He used to say, "Never trust the Irish" – followed by that grin.

So, I helped him to the toilet, to take off his clothes, to dress him, to give him his showers and to prepare his food. He was unable to put shirts on over his head, so I bought shirts that buttoned in the front. He could not always remember how to put his arms in his sleeves. I stopped giving him his hearing aids, because I caught him in time just as he was about to eat them. He was agitated most of the time – so was I.

ೲ ೞ

I had read that pets could be calming. Certainly we needed something peaceful. Should we have another cat in our lives? When I suggested the idea to Jim, he became upset.

Jim's world seemed Orwellian, Kafkaesque, hierarchical and bureaucratic. We couldn't just get a cat; we had to abide by rules, and that woman in the front room of the apartment seemed to be part of a regulatory staff. 'Cat acquisition' apparently required authorization. So, as our neighbor had in Lenox, when Jim didn't believe he had the right to be in his own apartment, I produced the condo by-laws and sat down with him to discuss the matter formally. I showed him the sentence that said pets were permitted. I didn't know if he could read the line I showed him, but he acceded to my request.

As a result, we went to the Humane Society and picked out Cleo. When we brought her home, Jim was not interested in her at all. In fact, he shoved her away when she came near or if she jumped up onto the ottoman near his feet.

But Cleo turned out to be therapy for me, because she gave me something to smile at and to worry about besides Jim. Unfortunately, Cleo awakened at 4:00 am, sometimes only minutes after Jim had fallen asleep, so I was weary. She became visibly ill one Christmas Eve. Although the vet tried to save her, he couldn't; she died. She was a sweet, warm friend I could hold, when I could no longer hug my husband.

Cleo's death seemed to be another reminder of illness, loss and death: Jim, Mom, Dad, a colleague in Ireland, Liam, and a friend, Fran, even Ellen's move to Portland, Oregon. Tears came to my eyes when I opened a letter from Ellen with a photograph of my two grandchildren. I steeled my heart. Cleo's death seemed unfair. In football, I think the term is 'piling on.'

A year later without Jim's input, I decided to get another cat. When I brought her home, she cried for two hours, so I called the Humane Society and said sadly, "Please keep the donation, I'm bringing her back." An unhappy cat and a demented husband were more than I could handle, so I bought some fish thinking Jim might enjoy their color and movement; he didn't look at them or couldn't see them. They lived.

Choosing an older cat had been a wise decision because an energetic kitten might have added to his hallucinations. Jim had begun seeing small creatures on the floor or in the corners of the rooms. I stepped on the spot he was staring at or said that "whatever" he saw was not there. He talked to people he must have seen sitting in chairs or standing in corners. I was inept at handling them, too.

By now we were unable to have conversations about the weather, getting a cat, eating a sandwich, taking a walk, getting the mail, putting gas in the car or having toast. His condition was beyond my comprehension and my skills.

As the days of confusion mounted, I asked myself, would I ever remember the good times? Which part of our lives together was the fantasy? Which the reality?

සා ද

Increasingly tired and lost, I learned that the local Alzheimer's organization had a daycare program, so I met with the director who suggested, "Let Jim believe he is volunteering to help out on the program." On the day we tried it out, eight other dementia sufferers were present. We arrived, and we all sat in a semi-circle, as the facilitator explained the information she had written on a white board. She had printed the day, the date and had drawn a picture of a sun with a smiley face, to describe the day's weather. When she took attendance, two people argued over which of them was nicknamed 'Captain Joe.' Within minutes of our arrival my brilliant educational guru said, "What are we doing here? Let's get out of here." He reached for my hand and was out of his chair heading for the door.

Jim was an educated, intelligent, confused, paranoid, hallucinating, delusional man, not a kindergartener – so much for daycare.

Although the program didn't work for Jim, and the social worker's advice at the support group meetings provided me with little help, I respected the director. One day, in utter desperation, I went looking for her. I found her as she was just finishing a meeting with the Director of Nursing from the local technical college. I waited. When I saw them, I blurted out, "Please, please, I need to talk. I am losing my mind."

They sat me down and said, in no uncertain terms, "You cannot take care of Jim by yourself anymore." They asked a simple question: "If you break down, if your health deteriorates, what will happen to Jim?" I didn't want to believe it or hear it, but I knew in my heart they were right. I had to acknowledge that I couldn't go it alone anymore. I had to get help, but how could I admit to myself that I couldn't help him?

The diagnostic process itself had been emotionally draining. We had seen physicians, had names of diseases and had tried medications, but I had no insights into the awful and dramatic behavioral changes that his illness had already wrought and would continue to make, and I didn't know how to handle them anyway. I was naïve to think I could help him; my ignorance seemed to make things worse, and I was worn out.

The notion of bringing in help was earth-shattering to me. That I was incapable of caring for the man I loved was nothing short of failure – of unfathomable proportions. I loved Jim and had let him down in his hour of greatest need. I simply wasn't up to the task. What an admission! What guilt!

When I left the two women, I phoned a friend to tell her what they'd said to me. She listened and then quoted the airlines, "Put your oxygen mask on yourself first, then on the person next to you." I understood what that statement meant. To protect him, I had to protect me; I returned home with a heavy heart. I had no idea what "getting help" meant, or how it would change our lives. All I understood was that I couldn't go it alone anymore.

సౌ ಲ

Because I had seen how hard it was to protect my mother from losing her assets when my father became ill, we had purchased long-term care insurance – fortunately. When my parents were both unwell, we had talked to a lawyer and our accountant to determine how to handle Mom's situation. When Jim and I selected our insurance, to keep our premiums down, we had bought a three-year plan with a 100-day deductible. We did so based on statistics; at that time, people usually went from hospital to nursing home, as my mother had, and Medicare paid up to 100 days. According to the Center for Disease Control and Prevention, the average length of stay in a nursing home in 2004 was 835 days, shorter than the lookback period, the time when you can divest yourself of your assets. It was a good decision – when we made it.

Ironically, my decision to continue driving south seemed to have been a wise one, not only because of the weather and the space in the apartment but also because the daily reimbursement from the insurance company was better suited for the costs of help in the South than in the more expensive Northeast.

After a couple of days of thought, defeated and resigned, I found the telephone number of the insurance company and called to ask what I had to do to activate our policy and how to use the money.

I had already learned from our sojourn at the skilled nursing home that Medicare didn't necessarily pay the first 100 days, and Jim would not be coming off a hospital stay. The representative explained that the company required a nurse's evaluation of Jim, so she arranged for someone to come over. When she arrived, she asked Jim questions which he couldn't answer. He did know his name and his birthday. He didn't know his address or the answers to anything else she asked. Afterwards, she looked at me sadly and asked, "How have you been managing?" What was there to say? Badly?

Jim was approved, his insurance activated. But what was it for? My choice was either to bring people into the house or go to a nursing facility. I knew we would be bringing help into the house.

As I anticipated, we had to pay the 100-day deductible out-of-pocket from our savings. The representative at the insurance company explained that we had to hire certified nursing assistants (CNAs) from a licensed agency or have licensed people care for Jim.

I went to the yellow pages of the phone book and found the listing for local home health agencies. I phoned and explained that I needed help during the day for a man with probable Lewy Body Dementia. I would be the night shift, as I would be throughout his illness. Having help during the day meant that I could leave him and not worry, and I would have some relief. That was that!

While I learned the hourly rate, I hadn't a clue what the real 'costs' were, what the aides' training was, or what the implications of having strangers in our home would be. I simply hadn't thought about it. All I knew was that I needed help! What a disaster!

When I made contact with the agencies, I made a number of assumptions, the first of which was that the agencies were in the business of caring for people with all manner of illnesses and knew how to handle them. As a consequence, I had no questions. They asked me when I wanted help and for how long. I hadn't even thought about the timing until they asked, so I said, "8:00 am to 4:00 pm, seven days a week." That would change, because I would need help feeding him, changing him and putting him to bed.

Only one representative of an agency offered to visit me and to meet Jim. When she came over, Jim was walking around the living room pushing the hamper, a silly gift I had bought him years earlier since he was the 'laundry guy.' In his current condition, though, he often shoved it against the door to keep people out of the bedroom. This woman said, "If an illness like Jim's were to strike my husband, I would be 'outta' there." Wow! At least she came over. The other agencies took the information over the phone. I couldn't use the assistance of the woman who visited us because her agency didn't employ 'licensed' people; they provided companions – again, my learning curve.

As I said, when I told the agencies that Jim was suffering from Lewy Body Dementia, I assumed they were familiar with the disease and how to deal with it, even if I didn't. After some bitter experiences, I learned not to assume.

Therefore, I assumed that the aides – mostly women – who were sent to care for Jim were trained to deal with dementia, and I was entrusting them with the most precious man in my life – no different from any new mom leaving her child with her first babysitter. What a revelation!

Yes, as I saw it, they were trained – to complete timesheets, to get them signed and to turn them in on time at the agencies. Aides arrived late or left early to "drop off their time sheets." The first aides who came to 'help' did not know how to handle

Jim, so I found myself morphed from the weary wife of a deranged man into a mother lion, bear or alligator protecting her helpless young from apathy and incompetence. These people were not the skilled 'angels of mercy' I had imagined – far from it.

When an aide arrived, I introduced Jim, showed her around the apartment, pointed out what was in the refrigerator and what he liked to eat. I showed her his clothes and his closet, indicated where his supplies were, pointed out the bathrooms, gave her my cell phone number, explained his routines such as they were, described his personality, said he wore glasses, explained his love of books and music, that he used the word, "loo" for bathroom and "upstairs" for the bedroom. I also said, "If you speak slowly, he understands, if you wait for his response."

After approximately 45 minutes, I would get out of the aide's way and go off to do whatever I had to do, secure in the assumption that he was safe and well cared for because he had help with him. If this was a first visit, I deliberately came back within an hour or two to make sure that all was well, with the intention of going back out, if I needed or wanted to leave.

But when I came back, it seemed that my explanations had meant nothing.

During the first few months of getting help, I was stunned by what I saw or was told when I returned. Aides told me: "It's Jim's fault he isn't wearing any underwear"; "It's his fault he was wearing only a shirt and urinating on the kitchen floor"; "It's his fault he isn't wearing his glasses"; and "I tied his shoelaces together because he was playing with them." Another never smiled. Another said, "It's his fault he has no clothes on at all because he refused to put them on."

Was Jim on the computer in the front room surfing rappers' websites? Did he turn on soap operas? What had he been doing when an aide was asleep under a blanket on the sofa?

The aides were invariably on their cell phones, awaiting other assignments or dealing with personal problems. Jim was not the priority. And this was the 'help' I so badly needed?

Apparently the aides didn't have the skills to put his glasses on him or dress him or pay attention to him, and Jim seemed even more miserable and more paranoid.

The list went on. One aide talked to me and ignored Jim. I took her aside and repeated that he was slow in responding, but he understood what she was saying. She continued talking to me, not to him. At the lunch table she told a story of a drowning. I turned to Jim and asked if he had heard her story; he said, "Yes, it's tragic." She looked startled, so I took her aside again and pleaded with her to talk to him, not to me. She said, "Oh! You want me to treat him like a REAL person."

When I called the agencies to tell them what had happened or to explain that a personality wasn't a good fit, the scheduler let me know "I was being difficult." Once again, I was making assumptions. I believed we had choices. However, if I called to say that someone was working out well, "Oh, sorry, she isn't available. She's on another case" or "She is just available this week." I had become so distrusting, I was no longer sure that what they were telling me was true.

I couldn't bear to leave him like this, so I stayed home or went out briefly and returned. How could I leave him? What was the point of getting help?

One woman at an agency said, "Jim clearly needs to be in a nursing home because we can't find the right help." I refused to give up. I kept trying; some aides lasted a day, others for up to two weeks.

I encouraged the aides to take Jim out for a drive or for a walk; they did, but, in one instance, I learned from the manager of the grocery store that Jim had walked up and down the aisles yelling for the police.

So, the three of us went out together; at least I could accomplish what I needed to do, and Jim could stay in the car with someone to watch him, or they could take a walk. At times, we all went to lunch together or for a drive.

One young woman drove with us to Charleston when we went to see Jim's neurologist. Because her allergies were bothering her, she took an antihistamine and curled up on the back seat and slept. On the way back, when we stopped to buy bread, I took Jim inside the store and worried about leaving her in the car alone dead to the world.

On another trip a different aide came to Charleston. This time when we stopped for smoothies, I placed the order at the counter, paid the cashier, held Jim's hand, tried to carry the three large smoothies and find an empty table, while she went to the rear of the restaurant and read magazines. While I kept an eye on Jim and walked over to her to hand her a drink, I asked why she was sitting in the back. She said, "I wanted to give you space." Thank you. What we needed was a hand.

I felt optimistic when I was told about a young woman, who was "great," and she could live in, if I wanted her to. But I lost confidence, however, when she telephoned, yelling into her cell phone to get directions to our apartment – approximately 1,000 feet away from where she was calling. I concluded that it wasn't an ideal match, when she arrived at the door, strode into the apartment, did not ask to meet her patient, Jim, and said, "I ain't had my brefus yet. You got any pancake mix?"

Bewildered and frustrated, I called the representative of the insurance company and told her of our experiences. She asked me to write her a letter explaining the nature of the help we had been receiving, so I sent her a list of thumbnail sketches. As a consequence, they responded by giving me greater latitude in hiring; I was allowed to employ people privately rather than through agencies, and, if there were issues around certification, I could run the candidates' qualifications by the insurance company. For example, they permitted me to hire someone whose license had expired and someone else who was certified in a different state. By now I had learned that some agencies had 'umbrella' licenses, which meant that the agency, not the aides, had the licenses. I could not and would not give up hope of finding better trained, more empathetic people – and there was an upside. By eliminating the agencies and their fees, the insurance money might last a tad longer.

To find help on my own, I asked at the pharmacy. I called the hospital, doctors' offices and even asked at the bank. I asked a friend. Who do you know? Who do you trust? I discovered a network of caregivers. Once again, I was hopeful. But looking for people on my own had its drawbacks, too. I met a delightful aide who had written a Gullah cookbook, but she was rarely available because she was on the road promoting her book and almost immediately hurt her back in a car accident. I learned of another aide, but she was on another case. I met a woman whose current client was relocating; she was set to start, but she suddenly left town to drive to Texas to be with her daughter.

There were eight million stories and an equal number of problems.

I asked someone if she could come at 7:00. She arrived at 8:00. "I can do the first Sunday, not the third." "I can do the second, not the first." "I can only do afternoons." "I can only do mornings." "I am going away until …" "No, that number has been changed." "I can't do that Friday; I can do this Friday." "Sure I can work until seven." "No, I can only work until 6:00." "No Tuesdays." "I only do 12-hour shifts." "No, I won't work with you, if THAT person works with you." "I only work 8:00 to 2:00."

Then I met someone who considered sitting with Jim, but that didn't work when she said, "I don't deal with incontinence." I tried a retired nurse who "ordered" Jim around. Her approach was so authoritarian that he became agitated. I suggested she keep an eye on him from the porch.

I was introduced to two sisters who worked together and could cover for each other, but at the lunch table, when one asked Jim to say *Grace*, he muttered something, got up from the table and then whispered to me, "THEY are taking over."

It seemed to me that most caregivers had little or no interest in Jim and his likes and dislikes. While they would give him the food I left for him in the refrigerator, giving him his newspaper, engaging him in 'conversation,' or playing CDs of Mozart, Brubeck, Boyce, and Jarrett, which I left by his radio, was another matter – and forget National Public Radio's *Performance Today*.

I suspected that the programs that were on the TV when I came back wouldn't have been Jim's first viewing choice. That he was Irish, well-traveled and politically-aware seemed irrelevant, that he had a huge vocabulary and used periodic sentence structure that faded off into no object or subject seemed to be of no consequence or of any interest. True, someone was watching him and could phone me, but that wasn't the help I hoped for. No one seemed to try to communicate with him.

Eventually, eventually, umpteen people later, when my hope was fading of ever finding anyone who genuinely cared about the man and understood his disease, Carrie came into our lives. She was patient. She listened and laughed with Jim. She was physically and emotionally strong and understood the illness. She had worked in a dementia unit. She taught me.

Carrie would open the front door to let Jim's hallucinations out, saying, "I asked the person who was in the chair to please leave because he or she is no longer welcome here. They are gone now." It was Carrie who told me when Jim 'shushed' me that he had "been whispering all day." It was Carrie who was invited to take a shower with Jim, who laughed when he began to wash her hair as she bathed him. It was Carrie who was invited to use the toilet next to him when he sat on the portable commode. It was Carrie who brought him oatmeal cookies, who said he was on his 'ignore' button, who took him for walks, for ice cream, for drives to the beach. It was Carrie who paid attention to him, who gave him his books, who sat next to his chair, who talked with him, who listened to him, who played his music, who fed him, shaved him, dressed him, put on his glasses, his hat and found his wallet. It was Carrie who cooked what he liked when he wanted it. It was Carrie who suggested different clothing or different foods, who noticed a change in his condition. It was Carrie who called me when there was a problem or explained to him when someone was coming over to visit or make a repair.

And it was Carrie who became outraged and said, "Where is YOUR mother?" to a man at a restaurant, when he told her to "Get that crazy man out of here!"

Carrie sat with Jim showing him the pictures of our new car so that he would be ready for the change. I had been concerned that a new car might bewilder him. We all drove to the dealership, and Jim said, "This is where I get my cars." And he beamed when the salespeople greeted him with "Hello, Mr. Tierney." We got in the new car without a hitch.

We finally had 'help.' She cared for Jim and taught me. At first, she was only available a few days a week, but that was a start. It was possible. She was a godsend. Later, she became available Monday through Friday.

But even with the best of help, there were challenges. And Carrie couldn't be there 24/7.

ço ও

One of our interesting struggles was getting Jim a haircut. We continued going to our salon as long as we could. It was an outing. Jim would walk into the shop that we had been going to for years, look at Diane or at David, our stylists, and his face would brighten. He would grin and say, "Hi." After his haircut, after Carrie and I helped him out of his chair, gave him back his hat and glasses, he would reach into a non-existent pocket in search of his wallet; then we would walk to the car. Once outside, he would look at me as if I were a stranger and be unwilling to climb back into the car.

On other visits when we drove to the salon and he refused to get out of the car, Diane would come out to see whether he recognized her. Sometimes it worked; sometimes it didn't. Increasingly he balked, so she offered to come to the house to give him a haircut. The first few visits were fine, but then he shoved her. Diane bought us a pair of clippers for Carrie to cut his hair. Carrie also clipped his nails and continued giving him his one, two or three showers a day.

જી ભ

Leaving the apartment and getting in and out of the car was always a crapshoot. Jim might leave the apartment, or he might not. If he did, he might get in the elevator or not, or climb in the car, go for a drive and then get out. Or he might walk to the car and refuse to get in, or he would walk to the car, stand by the open door and then close it, or get into the car and refuse to get out, or walk to the car, get in, get out and stand by the door and refuse to budge; he wouldn't get in, and he wouldn't walk away.

The seatbelt offered another challenge; sometimes he held onto it and would not let it go. Five or 10 minutes might pass. Sometimes we offered him something else to grip, and he would release the belt – sometimes.

Once with Carrie standing beside him, I tried an experiment. Jim was standing by the open door refusing to budge. Always the gentleman, we had learned that he would wait for us to go out the door first. Was he waiting for someone else to get out of the car? I walked around to the driver's side and got in. Then I clambered over the console and climbed out the passenger's side. Once I was out, he promptly walked away from the door. When we wanted to leave, I reversed my trip; I got in on the passenger side, climbed over the console and into the driver's seat.

That routine worked for a while. My climbing in the car first increased the odds of Jim's getting in the car; however, getting to any place on time or at all became increasingly difficult, and Jim wouldn't wait. If we were going to a restaurant, once he was in the car, I would call ahead to order food, so it would be ready and waiting on our table when we arrived. Sometimes the order became 'take-out,' because he refused to leave the car.

When Jim held onto the seatbelt, we had to wait him out because his grip was powerful. So, too, when he grabbed our wrists; we were 'handcuffed,' until he was willing to let go. Several times, when Sylvia, another dedicated member of the team who joined us a few months after Carrie, sat on the floor beside him, she would ask me to get his drink or dessert from the kitchen, because he had her in a wristlock which always seemed like "Don't touch me."

One morning, he grabbed my wrists and held them for almost 45 minutes. The more I tried to extricate myself, the tighter he held them. I waited for Carrie to arrive. When she did, she distracted him and freed me.

∽ ✍

Unlike some Alzheimer's victims, Jim didn't 'sundown,' the term for increased confusion in the afternoon experienced by many dementia sufferers. In fact, he was more confused in the mornings. I used to think he was more agitated because he was still in a dream when he woke up. But what did I know?

One morning he hurried out of bed because he was frightened. I understood the words "murder," "victim" and "water."

Wondering about the cause of the distress was pointless. His morning confusion usually meant I was thrown out, grabbed, shoved, wrist-locked or "fired."

One morning I saw Jim grab Carrie by the collar of her shirt and hold on; then he grabbed her hair and would not let go. Carrie was imperturbable. She extricated herself from his powerful grip and walked away. She waited a few minutes and then walked back into the bedroom. She smiled. He grinned and said, "Hi! Oh, it's you."

ꝏ ꝏ

Then, we found dear, dear Bertha, who came on the weekends. What a sweet person! While Bertha understood the illness, she had worked in nursing homes where the clock established the routine. But Jim was at home to give him flexibility, to give him a choice. Jim got up when he woke up. He ate when he wanted to and had a refrigerator stocked with his favorite foods. He could shower as often as he wanted. If he walked into the bathroom removing his clothes, no argument, he got his shower. He could go back to bed or take the spread off the bed and lay it by the sliding doors.

On Saturday mornings, Bertha looked heavenward if Jim said "Hi" to her, as if to say, "Thank you, we are going to have a good day." No matter how damaged he was, he was still the boss. He seemed to need to be in control or tried to be in control of what little he could, and when he was upset, he tore sheets or blankets. Bertha was patient and understanding, but he could be a handful. Bertha was remarkable! She worked until the very day she couldn't work any longer.

When I went to Bertha's funeral, I was convinced that a Baptist funeral was the proper send-off – the singing, the wailing, and the agony, so different from Jackie Kennedy's appearing to hold in her emotions behind her black veil.

৩ ২

Jim was raised in Ireland as a Roman Catholic. He believed in God, but he didn't go to church, except as a visitor to the great cathedrals like Notre Dame, St Patrick's, Wells Cathedral or the Pro-Cathedral in Dublin.

Early in our relationship, Jim had said, "If I am dying, get me a priest." That remark was a directive. Jim wasn't dying rapidly; he was dying slowly from a neurodegenerative disease. Occasionally he said, "I am an old man," or "I am dying," or "I don't want to die." I remembered Jim's remark and thinking that it might alleviate some of his anxiety, I decided to talk to a priest.

Hilton Head had several Catholic churches, and the Director of the local Alzheimer's organization suggested I speak with Father McCaffrey. I mustered my courage, because I wasn't even sure how to make an appointment with a priest. I found the phone number, made the call, and, lo and behold, Father McCaffrey answered.

He said, "Can you come right over?" I said, "Yes," and I did. I found him intimidating, but also charming and funny. I explained that Jim was demented, what he had said to me all those years ago and that he used words like "dying" and seemed frightened. Father McCaffrey said, "This is easy. Tell him you met a priest-educator who will come over to perform the Sacrament of the Sick."

As I left his office, Father McCaffrey said, "May Yahweh bless you" and laughed uproariously.

I had no idea whether such a visit would serve any purpose, but I hoped on some level it might touch Jim, so I alerted Carrie to the upcoming visit. Carrie explained to Jim that a priest was coming. Bear in mind, we never knew what Jim understood, but on that day, Jim walked to the front door and locked it.

But later, when Father McCaffrey came, Jim sat in a chair while the priest got down on his arthritic knees, performed the sacrament and anointed Jim with oil. Jim must have understood something, because he repeated, "Thank you, Father. Thank you, Father."

As I looked on and saw Jim's tremors increasing, I suggested to Father McCaffrey that Jim was becoming agitated and couldn't handle any more. Father McCaffrey wanted to give him Communion, but it was too much. Jim was done, so the priest left. Carrie had prepared a snack for Jim, which was sitting on a dish on the kitchen counter. He walked into the kitchen with her, looked at the lox and cream cheese sandwich, grinned and said, "Is this Communion?"

I went back to Father McCaffrey's office to thank him and to tell him the story of the lox and cream cheese – which he loved. He told me that Jim was entitled to a Mass and a Christian burial and gave me contacts for the two funeral homes on Hilton Head. When I asked about cremation, he explained that it was perfectly acceptable, but he admonished me, "Do not divvy up the ashes among nieces and nephews; body and soul are to be reunited in heaven, and all the parts should be together." Even though we were having this dreadful conversation, Father McCaffrey kept it light, and once again when I left, he expressed his hope that Yahweh might bless me.

Father McCaffrey and Father Laughlin came back a few weeks later to give Jim Communion. Jim seemed bewildered, and I was concerned it was too much for him; I could only hope their visit helped.

After their visits, I visited a columbarium behind another Catholic church, but I couldn't imagine being buried with him in a Catholic cemetery. At the time I had become clinical and had distanced myself from the situation; there were no tears. I phoned one of the funeral directors whom Father McCaffrey had mentioned and drove out to meet him. He was a charming man who explained that much of his business was "shipping." He said people 'stop,' and it was his job to send their remains wherever they were supposed to go. He showed me a set of niches and told me to call him anytime, if I needed him.

I knew I didn't want to scatter Jim's ashes, although I had arranged for my father's to be strewn off Long Island. Dad was a New Yorker after all, but I regretted the idea that there was no place to imagine him – to think about him. I had the same problem with my mother. I didn't want her ashes in the ocean. A woman I knew said, "I want my ashes in the bunker near the 18th hole on the golf course because my family will always find me."

That wit I no longer had. I needed to imagine Jim in a place I could visit or visualize. Until Father McCaffrey's admonition, I had thought about putting some of his ashes in the places that he loved, but I didn't. I bought a niche for him and one for me, and signed on the bottom line. I forgot that Medicaid allows you to keep enough money to pay for most burial arrangements. Once again, I had been profligate.

Almost euphoric for having done something, I called my daughter in Portland and said, "Hey, you owe me big time." "Why?" she said. "I have just made our funeral arrangements." All she said was, "Hilton Head?" I guess you can't win for losing. I hadn't thought about it. What I knew was that I had dealt with the inevitable. That night, I actually dreamt that I was in the niche looking out at the view; it was strange imagining my remains where I had 'stopped.'

ശ ഉ

When Jim was unhappy with whoever was caring for him, he closed the door to the bedroom, moved furniture and then sat in his chair. But if he was with a smiling, patient, laughing person, like Carrie, he was relaxed and laughing too. But he fired everyone at some point or told them to "get out" or pushed them out the front door. Just in case, a neighbor made us a 'pick,' so we could get in the bedroom, if Jim wanted no more of any of us and locked himself in.

After Bertha died, we had to find someone else to help on the weekends. Again we searched, tried and failed. But we had met Sylvia, and she eventually became available. She too was patient and attentive but not as familiar with the disease as Carrie, so at first when Jim called her a "liar," she seemed to personalize his remarks as I had, but she learned quickly that it was pointless.

One day he whispered to me that Sylvia was a "thief," and I should "fire" her. We didn't.

By the way, Jim never learned names: Sylvia was Mylvia, Jennifer or Mary, Carrie was Marrie for a while, I was Sean.

Often, after Carrie had given him a shower, he would say, "Oh, it's you," or when I walked back into the room, he sometimes welled up with tears and uttered a full sentence, "I didn't think you were coming back" – whoever I was. At times, Sylvia-Mylvia couldn't extricate her hand at the end of her shift, and Jim would say, "Don't go." But, although certainly less frequently than with our first helpers, there were occasional notes in the log indicating that Jim wouldn't cough because he said, 'The French don't cough', or 'He slipped because he didn't want to bend his legs.'

ஒ ஒ

One Saturday morning, when Jim had reacted particularly badly after trying a dose of Seroquel, I think, now contraindicated for victims of dementia, he threatened to kill me. I called to speak to our neurologist, and the physician covering for him suggested we consider trying a special unit at a teaching hospital. I had never heard of it. He went on to explain that it had been created by a neurologist who had specialized in dementias. He had developed the unit to help determine which medications worked with individuals suffering from the disease. *Was there still hope? Had we forgotten to try something? Would something help?*

So, on Monday, I phoned our neurologist to ask his opinion. He said, "It can't hurt. Nothing else seems to be working." I called the unit and explained Jim's behavior to the social worker in charge. He told me that Jim would stay about a week to give the staff an opportunity to evaluate him and to determine what might work. I didn't like the idea of leaving him in a strange place at all, much less for a week, but our neurologist had suggested it might help, so I decided to try.

I desperately wanted to believe that the physicians in the unit could help, but I should have trusted my instincts. I had shopped for physicians but hadn't learned to ask for second and third opinions. I had absolute trust in physicians' knowledge of illnesses and medications, and despite their occasional interpersonal and communications skills believed they were careful and had taken an oath to do no harm. I was my father's and grandfather's daughter and granddaughter after all. And my Dad's conservative first prescription for almost anything illness-related was invariably, "Take an aspirin and take a shower."

At the breakfast table, I explained to Jim that we were trying something new because the neurologist thought it might help his Parkinson's. Saying "Parkinson's" was better than "cancer of the brain." Jim looked at me and said, "Thank you." I cannot forget the gentleness of that thank you. In fact, nothing anyone has said from that day to this has helped me forgive myself for leaving him at the unit; every day that I looked at Jim afterwards, I was heartsick.

Carrie and I labeled his clothes; we packed and drove, stopped at a Subway restaurant for lunch on the way and arrived at the hospital. The intake process included an interview. Because the questioning bewildered him, and he was unable to participate, Carrie took Jim for a walk.

I answered their questions, explained his behavior, his probable diagnosis of Lewy Body Dementia and emphasized his drug sensitivity. I figured they knew all that; they had the records, and they were physicians after all – at a teaching hospital.

After the meeting, we unpacked Jim's few things, put them in the dresser and bathroom of the twin-bedded room he would share with another man. Jim was wild-eyed when we left, and Carrie and I returned unhappily to Hilton Head. She made it clear that she wasn't happy I had taken him there. The facility was beige, cold, antiseptic, dimly-lit and decorated in metal and linoleum. For me, the physical appearance was reminiscent of *One Flew Over the Cuckoo's Nest*.

That night I called to find out how he was and to ask for their fax number, because I had typed up a sheet describing Jim's personality and his likes and dislikes. They had given me his patient number, so the next two nights, when I couldn't sleep and called to find out how Jim was doing, they told me what percentage of his food he had eaten and that he had participated in some "pine cone" activity. I was amazed. I felt hopeful. They told me I could visit him on the weekend. I brought him a crabmeat sandwich from Subway. When I arrived, Jim knew me and introduced me as his "wife."

But, on my next visit, all was not well; he looked awful. He was bent over and drooling profusely. One of the staff members told me that there had been some kind of altercation between Jim and his roommate. The other man was wearing Jim's belt, and Jim's glasses were missing. We found his glasses in the other man's pocket. The staff assured me that they were making headway but that Jim had been combative. I thought, "Take a demented man and put him in unfamiliar, clinical surroundings with strangers and have him lose his possessions, what did they expect?"

BUT I left him there. I called the neurologist and asked if he might stop by to see him. He did. Carrie drove up to see him. "I am a mess," he told her. I wanted him out.

On Thursday when I drove up to bring him home, Jim didn't greet me at the door; instead, he was sitting on a sofa all bent over. He was lethargic and wearing his hat. A social worker and a psychiatrist met with me and told me that they needed to keep him a few more days. I didn't know what to do. I told them he looked awful. They said he looked like that when he was admitted. I said, "No, he didn't." Apparently I was co-dependent and in denial. Feeling desperately alone and overwhelmed and not possessing the science of a physician, I agreed to a compromise and let him stay one more night.

On my first visit, they had pulled him away from the door; now he was compliant and complacent. On the drive back, I phoned the pharmacist and asked about the two drugs that Jim had been given: Haldol and Zyprexa, both antipsychotics. "Are they titrating the dosage too quickly?" she asked. I asked her the meaning of "titrate." "Trying to find the optimal dosage," she said.

When I got home, I phoned the psychiatric social worker we had met in Lenox. She said, "Let me do some research." I called the psychiatrist I had begun seeing. Both of them assured me that Jim would sleep it off and be OK in the morning. I slept fitfully. No one I asked seemed to know the effect of antipsychotics on Lewy Body Dementia patients; it didn't matter; the damage had already been done.

The next morning, when I was in my psychiatrist's office, he took a call from the social worker at the unit. He said, "Jim is being admitted to the Acute Care Unit (ACU) at the hospital. He is dehydrated, running a fever and rigid." I tore out of the office, drove too fast and arrived as an ambulance was leaving to take Jim to the hospital. When I saw him in the back of the ambulance, I was relieved to see that smile and that his eyes were clear, but all was not well.

ے ࢦ

When Jim was admitted to the ACU, a charming, red-headed nurse with an Irish lilt greeted him, and Jim looked happy. He was given Amantadine, to attempt to alleviate some of the rigidity that had occurred as a result of giving him antipsychotics, and he was being treated for possible Neuroleptic-malignant Syndrome (NMS), a life-threatening disorder that can be caused by reactions to those types of medications. Jim was treated and survived. He remained in the hospital over the weekend, while I slept in a recliner by his bed. I left him only to buy sandwiches, toiletries and smoothies.

But now he could not walk unassisted; he needed to lean on the tray table when the aides and nurses moved him across the room.

When I went back to the unit to collect Jim's clothes, a nurse did ask, "How is Mr. Tierney?" "He's alive," I snarled. By then, I had learned that had he not been treated so quickly, he might not have been.

Our neurologist visited Jim in the ACU, assuring me that the physician handling Jim's case was excellent. When Jim was discharged, he was wheeled out of the hospital with a 6" neck brace and orders for a walker. He wore the brace once — on the drive home. The physical therapist had stuffed a washcloth over the front edge of the brace to absorb the drool. Would it have been kinder if Jim had died that day? He had so little happiness in his life, and what little joy he had was taken away from him with his head bent over at close to a right angle.

Once we were home, I felt sick whenever I looked at Jim with his head bent like that. The man with those gorgeous blue eyes could no longer lift his head. The man who had walked erect, who had delighted in looking at the water, at the horizon, at dolphins leaping 30 feet from shore, the man who selected a condo that looked out at the intracoastal waterway, could no longer sit on the porch and see the view. The man who loved to walk, even in his demented state, had rigid legs and an even more inflexible body. The man who had slid into a bench at a Subway restaurant could no longer make that simple maneuver. He had more difficulty getting in and out of a car or a chair and in and out of a shower.

The once fastidious man now dripped food on his clothes. The first day he dropped coleslaw on his shirt was the last time he ate it. The man who still enjoyed eating broiled fish with a fork at a restaurant needed to eat finger food like fried scallops or calamari. If the food fell on his lap, dinner was over. He would get up from his chair and leave. Unable to tilt his head back, he could no longer drink from a cup or a glass. He needed a straw. He couldn't watch television. He was harder to shave. He developed irritations under his neck. He was unable to see out the windshield of the car or where he was walking.

Not too long after, we were outside strolling a bit and met someone we knew. Jim couldn't lift his head. I almost wept when he said to her, "Nice shoes."

He hurt. Only when he lay down did gravity allow his head to fall back. After a night's sleep, when he sat up, his head was up, and he could look you in the eye, but not for long. His head would begin to droop within a minute or so. At first we encouraged him to lie down on the sofa during the day to give his neck a rest. We gave him one-quarter of the lowest dose of Vioxx or baby Tylenol for the discomfort. We tried massage. We tried acupuncture. We tried physical therapy; the therapists recommended neck braces, but the collars frightened him, and the braces they offered were either too confining or too narrow to be of any use. And, of course, when a therapist came too near him, he yelled "Help, police."

One day when he was lying on the sofa, I said again, "I am so sorry about your neck." He looked at me and said clearly, "Sue the bastards."

With his head bent the way it was, he could see every spot on the carpet. One day I called to check in. Sylvia said with a laugh, "I can't talk now. Jim has me cleaning the floor." He saw every shadow or crumb. For anyone to talk to him, we either had to bend over or kneel down and look up at his face. If you stood next to him, with his head bent the way it was, he couldn't see who you were and frequently lashed out with his fists. Was this faceless body a potential threat?

Our neurologist tried different medications to undo the damage, but Jim couldn't handle medications. Any dose high enough to help might have created problems because of his drug sensitivity. Then our neurologist tried Botox injections into Jim's neck muscles. I prayed. I hoped. It was a dreadful procedure. Jim didn't understand what was happening and became frightened. The result of the injection? Nothing. Not true, his head sagged even more until the Botox wore off. In essence, Jim was never able to lift his head and was more rigid for the remainder of his life. What we could do was try to make him comfortable.

కా సా

I bought a recliner, hoping that, if he sat at an angle, he would be able to see people's faces or the television, but he wanted no part of the new chair. Then one day Carrie noticed that Jim was beginning to sit in it, so she moved the chair near the television. Hurray! He sat in the recliner and could see the screen and our faces without our bending over and looking up at him.

Sometime later, the woman with the "nice shoes" gave us a splendid gift – her father's lift chair. Jim sat like a king, ankles crossed in his wonderful electric chair. What a godsend! As his legs weakened and eventually failed him completely, he could be raised to a standing position without our using our arm, leg and back strength to support him. Only Carrie and Sylvia were strong enough to move him on their own.

ഛ ഛ

I never forgot Jim's saying, "Sue the bastards." Whenever I looked at him, when we put him to bed or tried to find a comfortable position for his head, I was reminded. Why, oh, why had I left him there?

I requested his medical records from the hospital and spoke to our lawyer who took the records and gave them to a physician friend to read. He thought there was a case for negligence. This daughter of a physician was not only losing faith in doctors but was also searching for a medical malpractice attorney. Unthinkable! Finding a lawyer became a challenge, too.

The owner of our favorite seafood restaurant was stunned by Jim's appearance, and said, "I hope you are going to sue. I know a great litigator." I met with his attorney and gave him the records. After reading them, he said, "What you are going through with Jim's illness is gut-wrenching enough; you don't need to bring a malpractice suit." I thanked him and phoned another attorney. When this lawyer and his nurse-paralegal asked me to spell Lewy Body three times, I didn't bother to forward the records.

Then I was given the name of an attorney in Atlanta. He read the records and said it was a "state of the art" case. But when he spoke to a psychiatric expert, who said that he "believed they had done the right thing," the Atlanta attorney returned the records and suggested we find an attorney in South Carolina. I was given the name of another malpractice attorney; he was too busy, but he gave us four more names – one of which resonated with my attorney who by now had said I was "obsessing." But because he had worked with that fourth lawyer, he made the call and forwarded the records. The attorney read them and called me to say he would take the case. That call was what I needed. Someone had heard; someone believed we had a case. We were going to "sue the bastards."

Over the years, whenever a letter from the lawyer came in the mail, I opened it and put it in Jim's lap and said, "We are suing the bastards." Did he understand? I doubt Jim could decipher anything on the page, but I wanted him to know that I was trying to right the wrong that changed the quality of the remainder of his life. I will die hearing him say, "Thank you," when I told him we were going to the hospital that fateful morning.

Jim did not live to see the outcome of the lawsuit. In the end, there was no trial and no settlement, though the hospital wrote a letter of regret.

∽ ∾

After Jim came back from the ACU, someone suggested I consider hospice – for the help they could provide us. Even though I made the contact, when Jim was accepted by hospice, I was a wreck. To me, 'hospice' meant he was dying – an admission I was not able to accept. Hospice usually accepts patients who are expected to die within six months, and I wasn't prepared for that. In fact Jim didn't die in six months but lived four more years.

Hospice assigned a nurse to Jim. Once every week or so, she came over, took his blood pressure, checked his vital signs and chatted with him. One day when she sat with him, he said, "I am worthless," and he cried. She tried to reassure him that he wasn't and held his hand.

On one visit, the nurse suggested we try a hospital bed because it would be easier to get him to a sitting position. Through the magic of hospice, they arranged for the bed. Jim sat in it. He laughed, but Jim was unsteady and still ambulatory, and we worried about his knocking into the crank and the metal corners, and the mattress was thin. The bed was out of the apartment in 24 hours – also the magic of hospice. We had already asked a neighbor to sand down the corners on the dresser and bedside table for fear that Jim might hurt himself if he fell.

While we still were working with the attorney in Atlanta, he called to ask that Jim have an EMG, electromyography, a test for the health of muscles and nerves. I didn't want to put him through any tests, but if we were to proceed with the lawsuit, we had to do it. However, once you belonged to hospice, you belonged to hospice. They owned the patient, so I called to check with them and explain that we needed to arrange for the EMG. Jim was instantly discharged. Hospice seemed concerned that this test might lead to more tests, an audit and maybe a refund of Medicare money.

What! I called someone I knew who was the former head of a hospice. I asked her how they could talk about my husband like this. He was not a number! He was a person, my husband, who needed a test. At my friend's suggestion, I called the executive director of the hospice and explained that although I understood organizations, they should consider Jim as an individual, as a person – my ongoing struggle. The director apologized and said, "We will always be there for you, and Jim can be readmitted anytime."

Prior to his discharge, I called them on two other occasions. I had tried to reach our nurse at 8:30 one morning and was told she was away. I asked if they could send someone else, because

Jim had awakened in a pool of diarrhea and was gagging and had the hiccups. Clearly, he was sick. They promised to call me back. In the meantime, Carrie cleaned Jim up; I called a doctor, who prescribed Thorazine. We gave Jim small amounts of fluid. I went to the pharmacy to pick up the prescription and asked the pharmacist what Thorazine was. I had finally learned to ask! The reply, "Thorazine is an antipsychotic." No! Apparently, one of its side effects is that it stops hiccups. I left the bottle on the counter.

The pharmacist suggested we try an over-the-counter antacid, Gaviscon. While I took it, we didn't even need to use it, because Sylvia had tried her magical ear remedy which successfully stopped his hiccups; Jim ate a bit and appeared to be feeling better.

At 5:00 pm, the phone rang. It was someone from hospice. "Sorry about not getting back to you sooner; we were busy. Why don't you take him to the doctor?" "Thank you very much," I said, "we handled it."

The next time I had occasion to speak to our neurologist, I told him about the prescription for Thorazine for hiccups. He said, "It's a good thing you didn't give it to him; it would have turned him into a pretzel."

I called hospice one other time, because Jim had fallen trying to get out of bed. Hospice recommended that I call Security. As previously when he didn't know his own apartment, the guards were remarkable. They came over, picked him up and put him in bed.

Sometimes, at night, if Jim's legs buckled under him, or he slid onto the floor, and I couldn't get him back up, I called them. While we waited, Jim would lie peacefully on the floor with a blanket over him and a pillow under his head. I told him help was on the way. He would laugh when the guard helped him up and once actually said, "Thank you, Officer." Security was there for him.

While we belonged to hospice, I was invited to meet their new pastoral counselor, a gracious lady, with that same social work voice. We met for coffee; I felt a whole lot better when she explained I was suffering from "anticipatory grief." I had a label for my heartache. I had already seen their social worker and his offer of "hugs" didn't help.

To come to terms with my own pain and with Jim's disappearance, I did attend a bereavement group that hospice organized. I had needed special dispensation because Jim was alive, even though he could no longer discuss the day's events, offer his views on local politicians, tell me if he liked my new haircut, say that he needed new batteries for his hearing aids, laugh at my neuroses, or be willing to "smooth my feet, please." Having to walk into a church for the meeting was difficult, but I was looking for solace. I felt guilty having a living husband, but it helped being around other people in pain.

The other folks in the bereavement group graduated. I didn't. The facilitator expressed her hope that a couple from the group would marry. I finally wearied of the meetings after several men cited Scripture to justify their desire to meet women, and when one young woman said in her first week, "My husband's death was the most beautiful experience of my life." In week two she was "angry at God," and in week three she asked, "Is this the proper forum to talk about dating?"

৵ ৶

I was walking on a treadmill at a gym when I recognized someone from the bereavement group. We struck up a conversation. He had lost his wife, was feeling lonely, and he admitted he was uncomfortable doing anything on his own. I told him I went to the movies on Fridays, as Jim and I always had, and I said he was welcome to join me.

We met in the lobby of the theatre, went Dutch but sat together. We said nothing to each other and parted after the credits. At subsequent meetings at the gym, I kept him apprised of the latest cultural events. He told me his sister-in-law was in town and hoped I would join them for lunch. I had been invited to a couple of Christmas open houses, but I usually left after about 30 minutes or so, because I knew no one, had few conversational gambits, little holiday spirit and was paying out-of-pocket for Sylvia to stay an additional hour in the evening. Going out to lunch was no problem, so I accepted the invitation to join them and thought nothing of it.

A couple of weeks later, he invited me to be a fourth at dinner – his best friends were in town. I went but felt as if I were being interviewed. Then I received a bouquet of flowers. NO! He phoned to ask whether I would have breakfast with him because his daughter was in town. I declined. Then he phoned to ask whether I would spend the weekend with him. I declined. I thought I had been helping someone adjust to his loss, but apparently I was being 'vetted.' A few months later I learned he had remarried.

Jim was still alive and at times literally 'kicking.' We no longer made love. I couldn't remember when our lovemaking stopped, but, once in a while, he put his arm around my waist or suddenly reached out and hugged me, and sometimes at night he held my hand. Once he said, "Is that you, Lovey?" I think he recognized me. My husband was still there.

Using hospice was part of my continuing education.

By the way, whenever I used the word 'hospice' around Carrie and Sylvia, they cringed. Even though they welcomed the nurse's visits, they didn't feel that hospice was what Jim needed. I think they associated it with death rather than life.

I hadn't moved our records from our last internist, so I made an appointment hoping the doctor might be able to offer the name of someone. When I explained why I was there, no names were forthcoming. Instead, the response was amazement that I was still trying to care for Jim and that his developing aspiration pneumonia would be a good thing.

I moved our records.

⤳ ⤴

Six years after Jim's diagnosis, we had two devoted aides in place, but we needed a backup, because they were not always available. Carrie came Monday through Friday during the day, and Sylvia arrived at the end of the day to give Jim his dinner and put him to bed. She worked some weekends, but two people were not enough. And Bertha was gone.

We searched for people in case of emergency, for holidays, for difficult days of the week. It was an onerous task, and we needed someone who would work well with Sylvia and with Carrie. So we looked again, and Carrie or Sylvia worked with each new person to explain Jim's routines and care.

I was referred to an aide who was studying to be a Licensed Practical Nurse (LPN). She had fixed views of her own about how to care for Jim and did not work out as part of the team. Another thought I needed a vacation; six weeks later she phoned out of the blue and told me that I should not leave my husband in the care of strangers. Another made it clear that if she did not like the job, she would not stay. She arrived an hour late on her first day, maintaining it was my mistake.

I told another aide I would pay her a fee to 'shadow' Sylvia for a few hours. She came; she shadowed. It was Valentine's Day, and I happened to have a little charm bracelet to give her daughter. Everything seemed to go well, but then she called and said I had promised her a different rate. I had told her two rates: one for the time she shadowed Sylvia and the other when she was on her own. Feeling I was being called dishonest, I figured we were getting off to a poor start and did not pursue her returning.

We tried another aide. She seemed sweet and enthusiastic, but she was in such a hurry to get to her second job, she rushed Jim from his recliner to his chair. Jim always needed to be told what was happening. Putting him to bed typically took 10 to 15 minutes. She tried to accomplish it in less time, but by hurrying she lost time. Jim became livid. He said, "Sit. Stay there." Even though he was in his chair and his limbs were stiff, he grabbed her hair and kicked her as she leaned down to adjust his feet. Then his hands went for my throat. I moved – quickly. I felt sorry for her. She was in tears. After he calmed down, we got him into bed. She was late for her second job and decided against returning to us.

Eventually, we met Denise, who came on those afternoons when Sylvia couldn't come, but she was older and not as strong, so we usually did the transfers together. One weekend she fell at home and broke a rib, so while she recuperated, once again we had to keep our eyes out for someone else. Occasionally, I would recruit a friend just to come over to help me get him into bed. By and large, we had a team, but it was nerve-wracking, because other people's schedules seemed as fragile as Jim's health was.

ᔑ ᔐ

Once I felt secure leaving Jim, I knew I needed to find ways to distract and help myself. The support groups hadn't worked, and hugs and labels weren't meeting my needs.

I needed a therapist or counselor to talk to about my fears – my life. I needed to find someone to whom I could express my feelings when Jim said, "You deserve better," when he managed to put a knife in a bottle and painstakingly spread mayonnaise on some bread, when he held open a Ziploc bag I gave him and let me fill it with Fig Newtons, or when he put a dirty dish in a cabinet or actually walked toward the sink with a dish in his hand.

Just as it had been when searching for doctors, aides and lawyers, it took more than one visit to find the right person: therapist, psychologist, psychiatrist – it didn't matter. I needed to talk. I saw a psychologist. We talked about my getting involved in tennis and tennis tournaments and the frustrations of dealing with insurance problems. I didn't play tennis and had little interest in insurance companies.

Another counselor was empathetic and generous. I sank into the pillows on the sofa, and was encouraged to have a glass of wine in the evening, to take luxurious baths and long walks on the beach; I barely had time to brush my teeth and shower.

Another therapist leaned back, hands on head, feet on a coffee table, and "concurred" that support groups weren't helpful. I sensed we needed more room in the office for our respective egos.

Eventually I met a calm, empathetic, practical psychiatrist. At our first meeting, I asked, "Do you still do 'talk therapy,' or do I have to take drugs?" He grinned and said, "I think I still remember how talk therapy works." He helped me hear Jim's voice. He frequently asked, "What would Jim have told you to do?" Jim believed in me. In the past when I was filled with self-doubt before I gave a talk, I heard Jim scold me for my feelings of inadequacy. "Of course, you can do it." But now, did I even want to?

Periodically, my psychiatrist offered me antidepressants, like Celexa or Lexapro, and I humored him by trying a pill or two, but Jim's experience militated against any affection for drugs, and I stopped immediately if headaches began, which they did. However, when he recommended fish oil for depression, I took it. I avoided prescription drugs. I tried Sam-e and melatonin. If I had known some Native American dances or had voodoo charms, I would have tried them, too.

I continued taking yoga classes and trying to "breathe." At times they worked; at other times I just curled up in a ball on the mat.

I tried acupuncture. The acupuncturist put some needles in my hands and in my calves, and I felt an electric shock from one foot to the other. I felt stronger when I left his office. Placebo effect? Who knows? Was I better able to accept Jim's outbursts, his shredding, lifting a spoon to feed himself, taking a crust of bread and using it like a spoon, putting the handle of a fork to his lips and sipping from it, or trying to eat a napkin? I went back for more.

We took Jim to the acupuncturist to see if it might help his neck. But getting there involved all the obstacles that leaving the house required. Would he leave, would he get in the car, would he get out, would he enter the hallway to the office? Sometimes he did, and he would take off his hat and glasses slowly and extend his hand and say, "Hello, Richard." Whether it helped or not, there was no way of knowing, but Jim allowed 'Richard' to massage his neck, and, afterwards, we would leave for lunch – IF all the variables worked in the reverse order. Finally, Jim wouldn't leave the apartment, so I continued the treatment on my own.

"What a beautiful day!" the acupuncturist said. "I hear that it is supposed to rain tomorrow," I said. He grinned, "All I care about is today." He encouraged me to read Tibetan Buddhism; I did. I read the Dalai Lama and Deepak Chopra. I read books about feng shui, which prompted me to buy an uneven number of fish and put purple in my prosperity corner.

I called a psychic. The woman I spoke to told me I needed a break, a vacation, said I would survive after Jim's death, said his death was related to his chest and was connected to the number eight. She amazed me when she said, "Jim had four children." She said I would love again, live in the Northeast and cross the pond again. A tribute to my psychiatrist: when I told him I had spoken to a psychic, he never laughed or suggested I be committed. Instead, he said, "Different people have different insights."

Thinking that my educational experience might be of some use and that I might find something more meaningful to do, I went to see the headmaster of a local school. Part-time consulting? We talked about Yeats, Ireland and his desire to retire to a foreign country. Thirty minutes later, as I walked down the path, I could hear Jim laughing as he said, "Sweetie, what were you thinking?"

I spoke to a medium. She told me I should trust my intuition and accept the fact that, until a certain date, I would have no control over my life. Oh, and my parents said they "loved" me from the other side.

I saw a chiropractor, not for my spiritual well-being, but for the pains in my neck which were severe. She said, "You will be in a wheelchair, if you don't go to Duke!" My psychiatrist suggested I see a rheumatologist instead, who dismissed the "wheelchair" notion. He said, "Get a weekly massage. If you are in pain, come back and see me." I didn't see him again and found affordable massages at a local college. I also found another chiropractor, who adjusted my back.

I walked on a treadmill at a couple of different gyms because there were virtually no sidewalks in Hilton Head and walking on the beach was too painful a memory.

I discovered comfort food. At first it had been difficult to eat when I was taking care of Jim on my own. Later, I discovered carbohydrates: bagels, cookies, Szechuan noodles, lowfat Oreo yogurt with hot fudge, frappucinos, quesadillas, pasta. Broccoli and salads were for happier times.

I saw a rabbi, who said, "I can't do anything to help Jim." He spoke of the importance of family and encouraged me to read *Illusions*. I bought the book and read two pages.

Of course I still had to buy groceries and supplies, have the car serviced, phone the plumber, go to the bank, but with good, loving caregivers, I was no longer needed the way I had been. There was time for me – time I didn't want and didn't know how to use. I had always been happier working, and here I was on Hilton Head, and I didn't play tennis or golf and had no inclination to learn. When I had become restless in the past, Jim had always said, "Relax. Read a book."

ॐ ॐ

Thankfully, I had lunch with my friend with the "nice shoes" and told her that I needed something to do to feed my mind and my soul. She found me a part-time clerical job with a technology startup – which eventually failed. I made a few dollars, wrote and edited some articles and fundraised for them. I welcomed the distraction. For a few hours a week, I could change the subject and not think about home. At the office I was surrounded by an eclectic, hard-working, intelligent group of people, who thrived on one-liners and *double entendres.*

Some days, Carrie drove Jim to the office, and we ate lunch together. When I introduced Jim around, he managed to say, "Hi." Other days Carrie drove him to the beach, around the island, or to Wendy's for a stuffed baked potato. If I worked until 5:00, I hurried back. But one day, Carrie said, "Come home late. Don't come home at 5:00." I ignored her request until she repeated it more forcefully.

We picked a day; I dawdled at work, but I had nothing left to do. It was 5:15. I called home and asked Carrie, "OK, now what do I do?" I had no idea what to do with myself. She said, "Don't come home." I stood in the office and looked around. What could I do? I hadn't planned anything. I couldn't create work. Finally, I had a brainstorm. I could drive to the Chinese restaurant, buy some take-out and bring it home. The drive would be 20 minutes each way, and, if I didn't call ahead, I would have to wait for the order. I drove to the restaurant, ordered some food to go, sat down at a table and drank some iced tea. It was well after 5:00 by now. I paid for the food, got back in the car and headed home. I walked into the apartment a little after 6:00 pm. I said, "Carrie, how did I do?" She laughed at me, and said, "I am proud of you." I went back to the Chinese restaurant the next day because I realized how relaxing it was to sit and eat. This time, I ordered spare ribs and ate them there while I read.

I began carrying a book with me everywhere I went.

However the next time I stayed out after 5:00 was harder; I had used up the 'pick up Chinese take-out' solution. What could I do? I didn't need groceries or supplies. I tried going to Wendy's and could only think of all the times we had stopped for a bite at a fast food restaurant when we traveled. I'd ask, "Do you want a 'fish something'?" And Jim would say, "Sure." "Diet Coke?" "Fine."

I was alone at Wendy's, ordering food I didn't care about, knowing that we would never again debate which of us would go to the 'loo' first. And when I went to the ladies' room, I had to take my handbag with me, because Jim couldn't 'keep an eye on it' for me. I was a wreck when I left Wendy's, but I dawdled and went home. Carrie's tests were hard because these outings weren't fun. Another time, I walked into a Cracker Barrel restaurant, and once again the guy was missing who would have studied the menu and said, "Grilled catfish with a side order of coleslaw."

౷ ౿

Jim was the loner, and I the gregarious member of the duo. I used to be eager and able to talk to anyone about anything. Ironically, during his illness, he was never alone and I was.

Having a demented husband was not the subject of scintillating conversation. Nor was I engrossed in hearing about other people's cruises, plans to travel north or dye jobs. I was boring and had no travel plans. That I got a better price for latex-free, powder-free gloves, changed Jim at 4:30 am, rolled him to one side without hurting my back or experimented with another stool softener weren't attention-grabbers.

However, under Carrie's tutelage, I became so brave that I planned a weekend trip to New York City, but the plans fell apart when an aide's schedule changed. I was relieved; I didn't want to be out of range if he needed help. Two years later, I took the train to Washington DC. I read all the way and stayed overnight. A year later, I took another trip and went to New York to see four plays in one weekend. His absence was palpable. My biggest gamble was a trip to Portland, Oregon. By then, Jim seemed to have no sense of time, so I doubted he knew I was gone.

ৎ৽ ঌ৴

I was still looking for things to do, not a career. During the last three years of Jim's life, I tutored international students at the local college, wrote articles for a local magazine and a Savannah paper, and taught some English classes at the technical college. When I became involved in theatre, I hung posters. I filed paperwork for a small company. A couple of hours a week, my focus was whether invoices should be filed under "MC" or "MAC." However, when the owner asked for my help marketing the company, I didn't have the energy for that kind of responsibility. I had had enough.

I took classes, attended meetings of the Foreign Affairs Association. I delivered Report Writing and Presentation Skills training seminars at the Marine Corps Depot at Parris Island. I proofread someone's autobiography and helped the director with the billing for the Alzheimer's group. I spoke at some caregivers' support group meetings in Beaufort and Bluffton. I went to the dentist, the post office, the pharmacy, the bank, for coffee and out to lunch. I edited online. I visited nursing homes. During the six months before he died, I gave two seminars: one in Baltimore and another at Camp Lejeune. I tried to keep busy, but it was sporadic and hollow, and I preferred to be near home.

I remained a fixture at the movies and read until the film started. If Michael Caine, Robert De Niro, Gabriel Byrne, Al Pacino, Liam Neeson, or Brendan Gleeson was on the screen, I watched watery–eyed. Why wasn't Jim sitting beside me?

After *The Magdalene Sisters,* I imagined Jim becoming misty-eyed over the images of the Irish countryside and heard him say, "I told you Ireland was a benighted country. You want to go back there?" The voice I heard was not the hoarse inaudible one he developed once he became ill.

People assumed we had intellectual discussions after movies – not so. Our reviews consisted of raised eyebrows, smiles, "Oh, well," "Well done," or "That was a disappointment" – like our reactions to previews: a whispered "Yes," or thumbs up or down.

I went to chamber music concerts. I could feel Jim's warmth through his tweed jacket as my shoulder touched his, but the seat beside me was empty. As I did at the movies, I brought a book and tried to concentrate on it, rather than remember sitting together at Alice Tully Hall, or rushing for a bus on Broadway.

For a few hours every day, I didn't see him fiddling with a fold of fabric on his nightshirt, handing us 'nothing,' or looking at the digital clock saying, "2, 2", instead of 8:22 or 9:22. The distractions passed the time, but they did not alleviate the pain.

I had two tickets to see Hal Holbrook in *Mark Twain Tonight.* I asked a friend of a friend if he wanted to join me. He agreed, but he didn't laugh in the same places Jim would have laughed. After the show, we headed down the stairs from the mezzanine.

The man on the step below me was wearing a blue, wool blazer – just like Jim's. Because I hated heights, Jim had always stepped ahead of me at the top of a steep staircase or escalator like the ones at Bloomingdale's, at Charles de Gaulle Airport or on the London Underground. He would turn, look up and say, "OK?" I caught myself wanting to reach my hand out to rest it on the shoulder of the man ahead of me in the blue blazer.

Why two tickets? It's what I had always done. I had to learn to stop buying two tickets. Would someone go with me? "Well, I'd love to, but I can't go that day." "Gee, could you change them for …?" "When?" "Where are the seats?" It was easier to go to the theatre alone and stick my nose in my book.

And people-watching was no fun anymore, and what happened to the nod that meant, 'It's bad; let's go." No more requests for "Two on the outside aisle or in the front mezz, please, unless the railing is very high."

I needed books to read; I used the library, but I had trouble going to bookstores, because I wanted to buy him the new Annie Proulx, Philip Roth, Robert Parker, John Updike, William Trevor or Booker Prize winner.

ཀ ༀ

Getting through holidays was always difficult; scheduling became a nightmare because all the aides had family commitments, and it was quite simply the 'holidays.' I learned to avoid malls. I spent one mild Thanksgiving Day reading a thriller near a hotel pool. Another Thanksgiving, I was a server at a restaurant that offered free dinners; however, it wasn't the 'soup kitchen' I expected. We servers appeared more needy than the diners.

Around Christmas, I bumped into someone who had been a server too. He was near tears. Apparently the "love of his life" had gone on a cruise with her ex-boyfriend and he was "dog-sitting." He asked if I knew anyone "beautiful and 40." What was he going to do over Christmas? I told him that I was going to the Chinese restaurant and a movie, and he was welcome to join me. He jumped at the chance. I could hear my mother," Do you pick up every stray?"

He called to confirm and said, "Wear bright colors!" What? I immediately regretted proffering the invitation; however, we met at noon at the restaurant. He told me his life story, about his ex-wife and his current love. But, unfortunately, the movie didn't start until 4:00. "How about coming over to my house for sex?" I said, "No." I remember thinking I should have said, "No, Thank you." Then he sweetened the deal and told me he had over 300 DVDs. We walked our separate ways.

When I got back into the car, I slammed my fists into the steering wheel. I was angry at Jim. I blamed him for this tacky moment. How could he leave me like this? If Jim had been well, then this stupid lunch wouldn't have happened. Without a doubt, Jim would have said, "You are such an innocent, what did you expect?"

Fortunately, my high school classmate was home when I phoned to wish him a Merry Christmas and to tell him what had just happened. I said, "I don't know if the guy was joking or not." Bill said, "The goal is one pass a week, and it doesn't matter if it is a joke or not. It counts." Thank goodness for Bill; I laughed, and I missed Jim. I counted my passes for the week when Jim said, "Hi, Sweetie," or "What a nice surprise to see you!" Or if he pursed his lips, when I leaned down to kiss him.

ೞ ഛ

Once I asked a doctor, "How can I survive this tragedy?" She said, "Think like a teenager." I hadn't a clue what she meant, but I interpreted her remark to mean, do what you loved as a teenager, or behave as if your whole life were ahead of you.

I had always loved theatre and acting, so, when I saw a notice in the newspaper for an audition for a community show, I asked Carrie and Sylvia, "If I get a part, would I be able to go to rehearsals?" "Yes," they said, "we will work it out." It had been years, but I auditioned and got a part in *A Black Comedy*. Because the reviewer generously said I was the "highlight" of the production, I continued auditioning and getting parts. Carrie and Sylvia, true to their word, "worked it out." I was in one play after another. Another kind reviewer wrote that I was an "acerbic Ouiser lovable and laughable" in *Steel Magnolias*. I had a blast as Eagle Eye Fleagle in *Li'l Abner*.

Because I had to learn my lines in the car, I preferred bit parts, so I was delighted when the local Equity theatre cast me as the crazy sister in *The Man Who Came to Dinner* and as the elegant Dolly in *Annie Get Your Gun*. I did dinner theatre at a local country club. I organized and performed in a benefit performance of *Love Letters* for the local Alzheimer's organization, and I had a role in *The Vagina Monologues*. It was fun!

Ironically, Jim had seen me deliver talks at conferences, but he had never seen me perform. I brought a program home to show him my name and picture. He looked at it, held it, put it down and applauded. Honest to God, he said, "Congratulations" and clapped his hands. However, when Sylvia played the video of *A Black Comedy*, he paid attention for only a few minutes. He said one word: "Depressing."

When I was about to make my first entrance in the first play, I took a deep breath. *Where was Jim and why wasn't he here? Why was I doing this? Why did I have to do this?* Theatre hours were tough. Amateur directors and actors were late, not so with the Equity folks. Rehearsals were almost always at night, and I got home at 10:00, 10:30, 11:00. Sylvia stayed until I got back. With a baby monitor nearby, I collapsed on the sofa for four or five hours and dragged myself through the next day.

At first being involved with theatre was sheer delight and distracting. Going to rehearsals meant I was way over my daily allowance from the insurance company, so I had picked an expensive hobby, and rehearsals were time-consuming. Initially I was enchanted by the sensitivity and creativity and loved working with the Equity theatre.

But after about eight months, I wearied of the off-stage drama: the actor who missed an entrance and justified it with, "I am bored." Another actor said, "Don't talk to me. I am bloated." Another told the lead, "You are overdoing it when you kiss me." A male diva was petulant with another actor, "When you don't say the line EXACTLY the same way, you throw me!" Two leads quit because they took umbrage at a remark about the Marine Corps. Another actor "left theatre" because he didn't win an award; actors were directing the director; a stage manager hated actors; an amateur actor was "sick of working with amateurs"; a director HAD WORKED in Washington; another HAD WORKED in New York; a director told us we all "sucked."

During rehearsals, I struck up a conversation with another actor who asked me what I did for "extracurricular activities." "Theatre," I answered. Did he mean bridge? Golf? Tennis? He clarified by telling me about his "strained" relationship with his wife. I added that to my classmate's weekly pass requirement.

I became friendly with a couple. When he was hospitalized, I sat with her. Then they decided to relocate. She headed north first, while he packed up the house. I offered him some empty cartons, but he called me one evening and said, "My wife is feeling fragile. She said to stay away from Dr. Tierney." I couldn't believe it. And my therapist worried that I was becoming isolated!

While I had found being involved in theatre an all-consuming distraction, I was losing my enthusiasm because of the added expense, the lack of sleep and the drama. I had read in my book on feng shui about "freeing oneself from physical, mental, emotional and spiritual clutter." I read that difficult people could be "clutter," too. I needed space from all the drama within the drama. I gave acting a rest, but not before I wrote a couple of articles supporting the local theatres.

I was trying anything to change the subject, but nothing I did took my mind off Jim and his illness. Absolutely nothing. Everything else was transitory. I tried to take it one day at a time to create meaning where there was none. True, I was becoming more self-reliant, and thanks to the acupuncturists, mediums, psychics, psychotherapists, massage therapists, Taoists, Buddhists, and mostly to caregivers and my high school classmate, I was learning to laugh – a little.

ॐ ॐ

I don't remember who told me not to cry in front of Jim. I tried not to, but I cried everywhere else. Are we born with a finite number tears? If they are limitless, then we won't use them up falling out of a swing, skinning our knees, or being disappointed by our birthday gifts.

For nine years, I had cried for me, for Jim, for us. If I failed to cry on any given day, then I made up for it on the next. I understand crying relieves stress. If so, then I was stress-free. I cried aloud or silently, for minutes, for seconds. A sob crept up my throat; my eyes welled up with tears. I took deep breaths.

The reasons for the tears were equally boundless: frustration, loneliness, helplessness, fear, anger, sadness, the loss of the man, a friend, a point of view, a sounding board, the dreams, the shared memories and shared experiences, the adventures. I cried because of his neck, his deterioration, physicians' attitudes and remarks. I cried when I hurt my back, when Jim took off his clothes in the middle of the day, when he missed his mouth with a spoon, over money. I cried because I was living where I didn't want to be. I cried when he said a phrase that touched my heart, when I looked at what our lives had become and at an uncertain future. I cried in disbelief when he lay on the floor instead of the bed, when he punched me, when he wouldn't get out of the car, when I couldn't tell him something funny, about a new restaurant or going back to Paris sometime. He couldn't say, "Keep going," or "Take a break," or "Have fun." I cried because I couldn't believe an illness like this was happening to anyone, and certainly not to Jim.

And I could cry anywhere: over the computer, in the car, in the shower, in bed, in doctors' offices, backstage, behind a shopping cart, in the bathroom, in the kitchen, in restaurants, over coffee, in the movies. I cried when I was alone and when I was not. I cried the first time I walked into a hospital or supermarket without him, or into a Paul Newman movie without his being there to say, "Not bad for an old guy," or "No, we don't need any blueberries." I cried when I saw him frightened by a new aide, when he was handled roughly, when he couldn't walk.

Jim cried, too.

The aides who loved him cried.

Dementia robbed us of a beautiful human being. When I asked my therapist who invented it, without a beat, he said, "Satan."

But I did learn to laugh, and I would never have been able to had it not been for Carrie's ability to see the humor in the madness. She and Sylvia and Denise and another new member of the team, Martha, threw their heads back and laughed or said, "He had us on the floor." They were not laughing at him. They were laughing at the impish twinkle in his eye. Even though he might have said nothing at all, they were ready for something mischievous—just like the old days. Until Carrie arrived, it was impossible for me to see anything except who he had been and what he had been reduced to; the comparison was excruciating.

But slowly I began to see the humor when he 'fired' us, or when I brought home a sandwich, and he said, "Is that the best you could do?" His voice was low, barely a whisper. Often the words weren't real ones; they were sounds or garbles of letter combinations. Sometimes, I was convinced I was hearing Gaelic/Irish. Then, in the middle of the garble, there would be a perfectly-formed grammatically-correct English sentence or a sentence fragment. When he asked me if I had quit, I was delighted and I told him, "I haven't." I smiled when he asked if I was divorcing him and said, "No, I am not divorcing you." When he suddenly announced that he "had to get to a meeting," I could reassure him that the office called to say the meeting was rescheduled. I learned to be happy when he asked Carrie, "Do you have a car?" I laughed when I walked in, and he was sitting in his recliner; somehow he managed to put his hands on his hips, and he looked at me and said, "Well, well, well."

One morning he looked at his breakfast and uttered, "Not that same mess again." Carrie and I laughed when he was watching *Gunsmoke*, and he suddenly said, "Good-looking jacket, but not my style." I laughed when he applauded during a soccer match or a football game – for no apparent reason. I smiled when he wanted to go "upstairs" or to the "loo," or when I heard him say, "Beautiful" while he was listening to one of the *Brandenburg Concertos*. When he put his baseball cap on backward, Carrie smiled and called him her "homeboy." It was lovely to see him hug Carrie, Martha, Sylvia and Denise.

When he hissed at me like a snake to scare me off, I could smile, or when Carrie told me he was "picking out a bathing suit for me" in the Land's End catalog. When the Gulf War started, there were three images on the TV screen, one each of Blair, Bush and Hussein. Jim shook his head slowly and said, "That schmuck." When Reagan's picture was on the cover of *Time*, Jim said, "Never heard of him." Carrie, Jim and I were in the elevator, and he suddenly looked at me and said, "You are an innocent, and she is just stupid." Neither of us knew where that came from, but we both laughed. I still do.

While I cried at the drop of a hat, I came to appreciate the magic of those once-off, once-a-day utterances. At times, I could say, "You are up to mischief," and his eyes twinkled. We handed him a glass with a teaspoon of Jameson mixed with water and ice, Jim said, "Cheers!" Like Jim's love-hate relationship with Ireland, I began to have a similar one with his illness because of my abounding joy in those moments and deep sadness for all the rest.

Carrie brought him treats. Sylvia brought him special Caribbean meals on the holidays. They phoned each other to make sure that they knew about any changes that occurred. They didn't miss a red spot or a scratch. They loved him. I was often out of the loop.

I had profound bouts of depression. I was tired of living like this and tired of living. I knew my job was to be sure that Jim was safe. I knew someday it would be over. And I was not prepared. I had no dreams of going to Ogunquit to have lobster roll without my best friend. I knew what the New York City streets felt like without him. And a flight to Dublin without his hand to hold? Would I be able to breathe clear Irish air without gasping at his loss? Oh, yes, I thought about Jim's dying; we would both be free, but I didn't see the future as opportunity anymore; I was waiting to get older, for my turn in the barrel, in a nursing home without my teeth, waiting to die.

PART FOUR

*Laughter is not at all a bad beginning for a
friendship, and it is far the best ending for one.*

Oscar Wilde

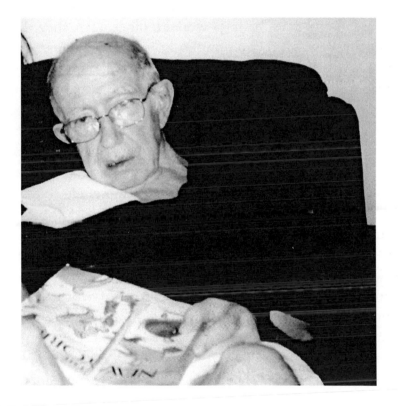

Five years after his diagnosis, I had accepted that I couldn't go it
alone and had looked for help. A year later, we had a brilliant
team, and I had begun to venture out. One would have thought

that life would have been easier. It was. But life became difficult in different ways.

We had a schedule – unless we didn't. Carrie came during the week, Sylvia on alternate weekends and at the end of the day after Carrie left. Martha alternated with Sylvia, and Friday evenings always required creativity. But the schedule was always held together by a thread. When Denise broke her rib, we scrambled. When Sylvia left for vacation, we maneuvered. When the holidays were coming, we planned months in advance.

As the months went by, Jim's ability to walk was severely impaired. Some days, his legs worked; other days, they didn't. Eventually, they failed him completely.

I hadn't realized that he would be unable to hold cutlery, to bring a spoon to his mouth, to feed himself, or that his tongue would tremble. In time he spoke in whispers in an unintelligible language. He was unable to bend his knees, to support his weight, or to lift himself to a sitting position. He would put a book or washcloth on his head like a hat, or position his glasses so that both lenses were on one side of his nose. He choked on food.

That he couldn't write hit me when I was cleaning a closet that had some boxes of papers and cancelled checks. When I opened the boxes, I was heartbroken to see Jim's handwriting on them, and then I found some file folders on which Jim had written "Social Security", "Medicare", and "Warranties." I saved a few cancelled checks and all the file folders. Later I met a woman whose husband had died, and I understood completely why she never changed the message on her answering machine; his voice was on it.

℘ ℘

Life was complicated too by the threat of hurricanes. Because the climate in Hilton Head is temperate, with the exception of hot, humid days in the height of the summer or a cold snap in January, Jim could be taken out in the fresh air – no snow, no ice. I could get around, and 'help' could arrive – no blizzards, no subway breakdowns, but Hilton Head is a barrier island, and we had the potential for evacuation.

Jim and I had evacuated twice because of the threat of hurricanes in 1996. We had booked a room, left early and driven ahead of the traffic to a motel in Macon, Georgia. By the time we arrived, every room was reserved. As people arrived, we heard about the traffic buildup on the island caused by the lines of cars filling their gas tanks. The police had opened more lanes leaving the island, but traffic crawled. So the thought of having to evacuate Jim in his condition was a nightmare. The hurricane season runs from June 1 to November 30.

Many people from Hilton Head choose to evacuate to Atlanta, but even when Jim had been ambulatory, we would never have been able to make the five-hour trip – he would have been too confused. Once he could no longer walk, we would have to maneuver him into a car, drive, move him into a hotel room and care for him – incontinence, feeding problems, bathing and all.

To discuss my fears, I met with the Emergency Management Coordinator and asked him what to do if we had to evacuate the island with Jim this ill. He said, "Don't do what so many people do – drive to Atlanta or Statesboro. Just get off the island." He showed me contour maps of Hilton Head Island. A major hurricane with a storm surge would cover it. I repeated what someone had asked, "Why do we have to evacuate? We live on the third floor." He explained, "Water is heavy. If windows break and water comes in, floors collapse." *Why had we chosen to live here!*

"Go to Ridgeland. It averages 65 feet above sea level. While you will get the wind and the rain, you won't drown." Ridgeland is only about 35 minutes west of Hilton Head, off I-95. It wouldn't have been a pleasant drive, but we could have made it if we had to. He added, "Go during the voluntary evacuation, or you'll be stuck in traffic." A 'voluntary' evacuation is what it sounds like; it is a choice and is earlier than the 'mandatory' evacuation. However, leaving early would mean that Jim would have to be away from his known world for longer. He may not have understood that this apartment was his home, but those surroundings appeared to be familiar to him. He seemed to have a sense of where his recliner was, bathroom was, or front door was. At times he pointed to where he wanted to go. And leaving for longer also meant more food and more supplies.

Prior to meeting with the coordinator, I had visited motels, including one in Georgia. I had hoped that by driving over to introduce myself and by explaining the situation, the hoteliers would give us a room before the rest of the evacuees from Florida or Georgia, but I had no assurances. When the coordinator suggested I go to Ridgeland, I drove up I-95 and visited a sturdy little one-storey brick motel. I was thrilled and relieved when the owners promised we could have a room if we had to evacuate. What a relief! During one particularly 'active hurricane season,' I made a reservation, and, as the storm track altered, I moved the date, then called again and finally cancelled. The owners understood and refused to accept any money for the inconvenience I had caused them.

Each June in preparation, I packed a box of food filled with prepared tuna, summer salami, Newman's Own lemonade, canned peaches, anything that didn't require cooking and left it sitting in the corner of the kitchen ready for a quick getaway. I filled the trunk of the car with a transport chair and bought extra supplies: Jim's underwear, wipes and gloves.

But I never would have been able to evacuate with Jim alone. One year, Carrie offered to let us stay at her house. But her family rotated care for her father, so the next summer was her turn. Then Sylvia agreed to evacuate with us, but in her case we needed to bring her niece and her godnephew, so we would need more than one room at the motel. One year Sylvia chose August for her vacation, almost the height of the hurricane season. Within days of her return, a storm barreled down on her own family, and she couldn't make contact with them.

Without the coordinator's support, I might have had a nervous breakdown. He would call my cell phone to say, "Don't worry" or "Consider the possibility of evacuation on Friday." He always added, "Don't worry until I tell you to." And, if I called him, he'd say, "Are you watching *The Weather Channel* again? I told you not to do that." I promised I wouldn't. I thanked him by writing an article in the local magazine.

Would we be able to get Jim in the car and drive to the little motel room? How would he handle being in a strange room in a hotel with thunder, lightning and wind? One year, when the outside of the condo was being painted, and the workmen had placed plastic sheeting over the windows, Jim became frightened by the strange shadowy figures outside on the porch. Another source of anxiety was the fireworks on the Fourth of July.

As Jim weakened, the hurricane evacuation worry changed. Would we be able to manage to move him in the transport chair? Would we be able to move him if he were lying down? I researched buying a van. But it was prohibitive to buy one in the case of one evacuation. I called a van taxi, but the driver said he had to take care of his own family first, and once he left the island, he would not be permitted to return. I called the hospital and the Red Cross. Both said, "Bring him." But, when pressed, neither knew exactly where their shelters would be and how they would move invalids. Ah, the joys of living on a barrier island with a man suffering from dementia! Fortunately, we were spared. But the tragedy in New Orleans taught us all that having a plan is imperative.

⋟ ⋞

If throwing out cancelled checks was hard, letting go of our king-sized bed was impossible for me. Even though we had had the 24-hour experiment with the hospital bed, thanks to hospice, I refused to give up sleeping in the same bed. The aides were not pleased with me. No question twin beds would have been easier for everyone, because we could walk around the bed to adjust Jim and his pillows or stand on either side to help him sit up. But every once in a while at night, Jim reached out his a hand to hold mine, and I was not giving up those moments – infrequent as they were. Sometimes when I reached over to change the soggy burp cloth under his neck, he would swat at me, but it didn't matter. We were in the same bed, I could feel his warmth, hear his breathing, shift a pillow, or move him if he began to choke.

In time I had no choice. We had to get twin beds. Carrie took the king bed. It had to be, because it was too hard to turn him, change him, adjust him, and make up the bed which had to be done at least daily and usually more often.

Actually those were some funny scenes. When he could no longer walk, we had to transfer him from the recliner to his transport chair to his bed. While Carrie and Sylvia could transfer him single-handedly, Denise and I could not. We could roll his chair close to the bed, bring him to a standing position, swing him around and seat him on the side of the bed, and lower him slowly to a prone position. But if we sat him down too close to the end of the bed, his feet would hang off the end when we laid him down. So, standing on either side of the bed using all our strength, we pulled him up by gripping the sheepskin on a count of three. On some evenings, Denise and I were drenched in sweat trying to pull him up, and we laughed with relief when we succeeded.

ço cç

While we didn't purchase a van, having sheepskins for Jim was just one of the many items we needed to buy. Sheepskin is soft and thick; it absorbs sweat, reduces pressure and wicks urine away. His illness was expensive; the aides were not the only cost. For us, Medicare covered only a few items. At least medical supplies were tax-deductible. To keep costs down I bought in bulk, comparative shopped online or set up automatic deliveries. I also took advantage of a $500 reimbursement for supplies or respite from a local advocacy group.

Jim wouldn't have been pleased by what we spent on him. For years he had scolded me for buying him books, a new shirt or sweater. One day when he was eating his mini-waffles with his fingers, I asked if he wanted more. He didn't respond. I brought him more anyway. He looked at me and uttered a phrase I hadn't heard for years. The last time was probably after I bought him a book that he had seen reviewed in *The Times*. He said, "I can't tell you anything."

To understand the costs associated with dementia, it helps to understand some of the symptoms: incontinence, swallowing, drooling or potential problems like bedsores. And, as Sylvia used to say, "You are damned if you do, and damned if you don't."

Like most of the drugs that he had been given, solving one problem invariably created another. For example, when we brought a transport chair into the house, it scraped doors, doorjambs or walls, which meant that walls and doors eventually needed repair. We also needed to remove doors. To make the chair comfortable and to avoid pressure sores, we bought gel cushions, pads and sheepskins. In other words, while we needed the chair, it created its own problems.

ৡ ঌ

Jim struggled with urinary and fecal incontinence. In New York, his overzealous bladder had become the focus of his attention. We were always on the lookout for a hotel or a store with bathrooms. In the South, we could drive to restaurants or movie theaters with bathrooms.

We had seen a urologist, but having a cystoscopic exam frightened Jim. The doctor recommended Detrol for an overactive bladder but said, "Jim's muscle spasm is so severe, he will require such a high dose that it will affect him cognitively." In essence, treatment for the spasm would affect his mind. "Damned if you do, ..."

While we bought a portable urinal to keep in the car, finding incontinence underwear became the priority. The type I bought resembled his former underwear. When Jim opened the first package, he said, "Thank you, my darling girl." Those pull-ups cost about $150 a month. I went to the supermarket or pharmacy and filled the trunk with bulky packages. I read the label, called customer service and discovered that the underwear could be shipped to us by the case automatically along with other supplies.

Jim had all manner of incontinence underwear. Some was designed for the daytime, some for nighttime. I bought absorbent pads, which weren't absorbent enough, so I bought briefs that were designed more like diapers, but the plastic irritated his skin, so I bought powders and creams to alleviate the itch. As he became more ill and barely moved, we bought mesh pants with pads, which were easily removed and not made of plastic.

I went online and researched other companies that could supply us with what we needed. Once in a while, when I was more depressed than usual, I would go to the LewyNet website. Long ago, I had ceased looking for cures and treatments. I did find an experimental study being conducted in California. I called and learned that IF Jim were accepted, we would have to fly out west and live there – and I could barely get him to the door.

ஒ ௸

When Jim stopped reading, walking and moving furniture, it pained me to see him sitting in his chair doing nothing, so I was always looking for activities to keep him and his fiddling fingers busy. Carrie asked him to help her empty the dryer or take out the trash – even when he was wheelchair-bound.

We gave him his wallet, and he would take out the credit cards and the money and stick them in the sides of his chair or up his pant legs. Sometimes Sylvia would order Chinese food and give Jim the bill, so he could pay for it. She always handed him the take-out menu, which he held upside down and backwards but still pointed to his choices.

I bought decks of cards with animal pictures on them. He would hold them and look at them and sometimes say the word that was printed above the photograph. His interest seemed to derive from the size and shape rather than from the image. At times he took two cards to bed with him.

When he said, "I have no money," I bought fake money and Monopoly money and put it in a plastic box. At times, he 'worked' on that for hours. Sometimes he gave Sylvia and Carrie money from the box when they prepared his meals. Before she left on one of her annual vacations, Jim handed Sylvia $500 in Monopoly money. Sylvia welled up. Despite the fact that she was an inveterate shopper, she claimed she hadn't spent it. We gave Jim washcloths to fold. After his twisting them, they looked like serviettes for a royal dinner.

We subscribed to *The New Yorker* and to *Time* magazine. We handed him catalogs to keep him busy, because he played with the pages. He crumpled them, shredded them, put them on his head or struggled to open them from the folded side. I bought children's board books, but they were not designed for an adult mind, regardless of its condition. I bought a small encyclopedia with pictures of dogs. He smiled and laughed at some of the photographs. I bought a fidget pillow from the Alzheimer's Store – no success. It had buttons and zippers, but he had no interest in it. I bought another that you were supposed to fill with water. It was too heavy.

For the most part, television held no interest for him either, until Sylvia discovered he could focus for a little while on black-and-white westerns. Then she happily found some soccer matches and track and field events, which he seemed to be able to follow a bit, because he applauded something – sometimes with the backs of his hands instead of with his palms. But, as he faded, so did his enthusiasm.

Then we had three great successes in a row. The first was discovering DVDs of classical concerts. What a find! Music remained. I bought a DVD of Herbert von Karajan conducting Beethoven. Jim was engrossed. I began to look for others, Nathan Milstein, other recordings with von Karajan or Neville Mariner conducting. I tried movies, like *The Sound of Music* and *Casablanca*, but they were total failures, so I bought DVDs of James Taylor, Barbra Streisand, The Chieftains, and the Three Tenors. His favorite was *Appalachian Journey* with Yo-Yo Ma, Edgar Meyer and Mark O'Connor. He applauded between numbers. I joined him and applauded with him. He watched that DVD over and over and over; tears ran down his cheeks, particularly when Alison Krauss sang. We always handed Jim the plastic DVD case to hold as if it were a program. He would hold it in his hands, lift his head a bit and seemed glued to the image in front of him.

One day, I barged in and said, "Hi, Sweetie," when Carrie had a DVD playing. He raised his fingers to his lips and 'shushed' me. If you disturbed him during a concert, as Carrie used to say, he put on his 'ignore' button. Several times after watching one of the DVDs, as he had with the soccer matches, he smiled, and brought his hands together as if to applaud.

The second success was at a children's store. I found a baby blanket with the head of a rabbit as the corner. Like Linus in *Peanuts*, that little blanket was always either in his hand or beside him. Another find was a $5 portable radio, which I discovered at a Dollar Store. Since his hands were always moving, would he be able to manipulate the dial? Jim played with that little black radio. Jim's busy fingers would fiddle with and turn the dial. There was static and whining between stations, but he actually left the dial alone for a few minutes and let the sound play. To Carrie's delight he might hit a gospel or country music station, and he would stop playing with the dial.

❧ ❧

Late in the illness Jim fell asleep as soon as his head hit the pillow at 7:00 pm. Most nights he slept soundly, but he had developed an unproductive cough. At night I turned him to one side or the other or tried to prop him up on pillows. Eventually we 'rented' a suction pump to get rid of the saliva that pooled in his throat. Medicare partially paid for that, but to keep the tube clean, we needed to buy alcohol wipes. One morning, he tried to drink from the suction tube as if it were a straw.

Sylvia positioned Jim; he slept on his left side one night and on his right side the next. At night, I removed or adjusted the pillows, so he would be lying at a different angle. We had little pillows, big ones, expensive ones and inexpensive ones. They were placed under his head, his arm, his side, a shoulder, his back, a leg, his knees and his hip. One night, he managed to press one over his mouth.

And as he sat and slept more, the possibility of pressure sores increased. When the body remains in one position too long, the blood doesn't circulate as well, so sores can develop on ankles, toes, elbows, or back. Left unattended, they can be ugly, painful and deadly. If anyone saw a red spot the size of a pinprick, they were on it.

၆ ၉

As his muscle tone worsened, his weight collected around his middle. We could no longer weigh him because, even with Carrie and Sylvia's strength, his legs wouldn't support him on a bathroom scale, and the price of a medical scale was prohibitive and seemed pointless. I bought bigger underwear, which was more expensive. His clothes didn't fit as well either. He had always loved shorts. Now we had ones with 34", 36", 38" and 40" waists, all with drawstrings.

The days of shopping at Saks Fifth Avenue for Joseph Abboud's microfiber shorts were over. He had loved the textures of different fabrics, and the days of the elegant clothes from Paul Stuart were long gone too, particularly when his cashmere sweater ended up in the dryer, or medicines or food dripped on his clothes. I used Land's End catalogs until I discovered Buck & Buck. He needed new shirts, sweaters and vests. We bought snap-backed nightshirts – lightweight and flannel, always in blue. Jim's feet were swollen; I bought socks for feet that swell as well as socks with treads, so he wouldn't skid when he was transferred from chair to bed. His old shoes were too tight; I bought shoes with Velcro tabs.

၆ ၉

When Carrie arrived, she started using a logbook. It was the means by which the aides communicated with each other about Jim. There they could keep track of his bowel movements and his food.

The section called Change in Condition might indicate that, "Jim has red marks on his back and waist. Heels and bunions red. Knuckles red. His bottom not as red as usual, but some." I added to that entry, "If you see a bruise on the top of Jim's left ankle, when I took the blanket off, his feet were crossed." Whatever anyone noticed was recorded and attended to by the next person. "Did he need another cream? Did he need to be adjusted differently? How did he get that scratch? What do you mean, 'He didn't move his fingers when you pushed his wheelchair through the door?'"

Another section was the Meal Log, which included the approximate number of calories, the time and the type of food he ate: one pack of oatmeal, half a banana, a whole quiche, his Starbuck's frappucino.

The Daily Log indicated how his day had gone and what they and he did. "January 8: Jim was awake when I arrived. I changed him. I asked him if he wanted juice ... Jim had a good day. Have a good evening, Sylvia with Jim and a good night, ET with Jim." Later, when Sylvia arrived, she would add, "Jim was on the way back from the bathroom, and he spoke to his wife and asked, 'What's for dinner?' and burst out laughing ... He was ready for bed at 6:50 and was out right away." Even though they called each other to find out how their day was going, that log was critical to them and to Jim's well-being.

And the log indicated what else we needed to do or what else we needed to buy to help him. I bought egg crate to put on top of the mattress to allow air to circulate and to vary the pressure points. Egg crate is not washable and has to be thrown away if it gets wet. I got a prescription for an alternating pressure pad (Medicare picked up part of that, too); it was hot and was like lying on an inflatable raft in the middle of a swimming pool. If Jim attempted to sit up by himself, he couldn't get any traction, which meant that his upper body muscle tone deteriorated. Again, you are damned if, … and Denise and I could not position him on that raft on Fridays.

We bought more creams and lotions for the rashes he developed. We bought synthetic sheepskin and put it on top of the pressure pad. We bought towels, sheets, blankets, pillowcases and bathmats.

ဗ ᴄ

While not enough can be said about what the aides did for me and for Jim, there was a cost, a downside to having help in the house. First of all, Jim was no longer simply my husband. He was their patient, and they loved him. One aide said that at a nursing home, the family stays out of the way and another wrote in the log that "there is nothing that I can do right." These comments made me feel as if I were 'in the way'. We are talking about four women with distinct personalities working closely together for almost four years – and me. They knew each other's strengths and weaknesses and mine, too, and it could become contentious.

One morning, an aide told me that I had better find Jesus. If I suggested that we needed to find backup help, then I was "threatening" or "underhanded." I wasn't changing Jim often enough at night. Carrie wrote a note to me and Denise, in which she was angry at us for our inability to take care of Jim. She wrote, "He can't defend himself when it comes to certain things but if it's not right I can defend him and I will. It's not fair to him." She wrote that note out of love for Jim. She addressed it to: "DENISE and ET." The lines among us were blurring; the boundary was no more. I had become another aide and a poor one at that. I was neither Jim's wife, nor their employer. Jim was always the employer – the boss.

I looked at the calendar with the schedule we maintained only to discover that hours were adjusted without my knowledge. One person announced that she had changed her hours permanently; one of the others would be coming earlier to cover. They arranged coverage among themselves because of a doctor's appointment or a family reunion. While I was delighted they were that responsible, they no longer considered that I needed to be, or should be, informed.

Nor, apparently, was there a need to phone me if someone was running late. I actually asked the newspaper delivery girl to wait with Jim one morning. I was teaching a course at Parris Island and was on my own; my calls to cell phones went unanswered. Was someone in an accident? Had a car broken down? Was it traffic? Meanwhile I made calls to arrange coverage. It worked out, but it was an extra strain if I had to be somewhere at a specific time.

I learned of the death of a member of Jim's family. When I told an aide, she said she already knew. I was dumbfounded. She had received a phone call from a family member and was told not to tell me. SHE GAVE HER WORD. She never told me. I was the odd man out. The morning I said I wasn't feeling well – it turned out to be a kidney stone – it was simply, "You had better see a doctor." Jim was the person they adored, for which I would be forever grateful, but feeling like a pariah in my own home was hard to take, particularly when I was expected to produce.

There were human problems: mood swings, health problems, cramps, PMS, increases in gas price problems, car fires, need for new places to live, doctors' appointments and money problems. We became one big dysfunctional family with one focus: Jim.

And there was sibling rivalry, too. Who did Jim love more? Who got a bigger greeting from him? Whose hand did he hold longer? Where did that scratch come from? Who was too rough? The log would say, "Jim didn't want to let go of my hand." Or "Jim said, 'Where have you been?'" Or "Jim didn't want me to go."

Because they loved him, because they took such good care of him, because I had gone through more than 20 people with little success, if someone was short of cash, I paid in advance. I gave extra cash when the price of gas went up. I helped someone find a new car, an apartment. I gave gifts, raises, bonuses, remembered birthdays and holidays – still my pre-nuptial job. But I drew the line at co-signing a loan.

I cannot find the words to express my gratitude for their love for Jim, but on some evenings I had to wade through two or three people who were sitting on the floor by his chair to be near my own husband because someone would drop by on the way home from another job. They had lived through four years of his illness and loved him, but I had lived through his illness for almost nine years, and I knew a tad more than they did about who Jim had been before. Like Rodney Dangerfield, I wanted some respect.

ও ৵

During one of my darker moments, when I was surrounded by women with strong personalities and equally strong opinions and was about to go around the bend, I decided to audit a course offered by the local college for people who wanted to learn to become certified nursing assistants (CNAs). By taking it, I believed I would learn to care better for Jim, to understand what CNAs were taught and to meet other CNAs, if I had to replace a member of the team. The insurance company picked up the tab.

The evening of the first class, when the instructor, Diana, started, I thought, "Oh, Good Lord, how am I ever going to get through this?" My classmates were young African-American women seeking to improve their job opportunities in hospitals, nursing homes, assisted-living facilities or private homes. There was one middle-aged, white man, named Rick, who seemed to know the instructor, Diana. *Did I look and feel as out of place as he?*

Diana began by reading the riot act to us. "If anyone is late, you will be locked out of the room." She showed us where we could go for a snack and added, "If you come back from the break late, the door will be locked. If you don't make flash cards of important words, you will be out."

I couldn't believe what I was hearing. *How was I going to survive this class!* I was being treated as if I were in junior high. I began to observe the class rather than be a participant. How could I be so out of touch with the education process? I didn't want to pay back the insurance company the $240, and I had told Carrie and Sylvia I was taking the class. They had congratulated me, and the college had accommodated me, as had Diana. I had to stick it out. So, I did as I was told. I underlined the sections of the book I was supposed to know for the licensing exam that I was NOT taking.

The first week Diana gave a pop quiz. A classmate had gone to the bathroom. When she returned, Diana told her, "YOU failed." Why? She wasn't there. I did too, because I only had a pen not a pencil. I was redeemed however, because I was wearing a watch.

Diana was determined to instill standards of excellence. Everyone was expected to be prepared all the time. She drilled us. She praised. She scolded. She taught us to use gait belts, to take blood pressure. If we forgot to put the rails up on the sides of the beds, we were ordered to sit on the floor. We were sent to the back of the line to "Do it again," if we forgot to sing "Happy Birthday" three times when we washed our hands in the classroom sink, or if we touched the knobs with our clean hands. The class was being offered near the Marine Corps Recruit

Depot at Parris Island; I thought I had missed the turn. But beneath the drill instructor demeanor was a huge heart.

One day Diana ordered us to bring our dinners to class – not surprisingly, they were all very different. She then divided the group into two: patients and aides. What she did to the patients! She put cotton over their eyes and ears; she duct-taped and gait-belted limbs to twist them. Rick was my blind patient, with cotton in his ears, so he was also deaf. He had on a straightjacket and was put in one of the beds in the classroom. A woman was made blind and deaf and tied into a wheelchair and then rolled deep into an alcove.

Then Diana announced, "No one is permitted to talk." She told us to come over to where all the dinners were lined up on a table. She randomly plopped food on the paper plates and handed us a small cup of liquid.

Then she repeated that there was to be "No talking." She added, "I want you to 'shovel' the food into your patient's mouths and NO talking!" I gave poor Rick his cold ravioli and peaches; he seemed OK, but when I put the drink to his lips, he grimaced. When we were finished, Diana told us to release our 'patients.' Then she asked them how they felt.

No one was happy. Everyone expressed frustration or a sense of helplessness. And the woman in the wheelchair in the corner? She said she felt "terrified." "I thought everyone had forgotten me." By the way, what was the drink? Day-old, cold coffee!

Her lesson was loud and clear. Diana said, "You talk to your patients. You tell them what they are eating. You reheat their food, or if they don't like it, you get a sandwich from the kitchen. You pay attention." I will never forget her class. I subsequently learned that, during the clinical part of the course that was held in a nursing home, Diana's students found a patient with a broken clavicle.

♀ ♂

One evening at the end of class, I got up the nerve to ask Diana whether she would be willing to come by our apartment, if her schedule permitted. I explained Jim's condition. Without hesitation, she said, "Do you want me to spend the day? I can be there at 6:30 am." I was dumbfounded. We picked a date. At first, when I told Carrie that Diana was coming over, she didn't seem eager to have her, but that reaction changed. Diana came over again and again, and she was welcomed.

But the first time she saw the bed, she ordered me to get boosts for the legs – that night! When Diana said, "Do something," I did, so I raced to a bedding store and bought them. At 9:45 pm, Rick and Diana arrived. Jim was asleep. While Rick lifted the head of the king-sized bed, Diana crawled under it and extended the legs under the head of the bed by adding the boosts. Jim awoke in the middle of the activity and grinned from ear to ear as the bed swayed like a ship in heavy seas. When they finished, Diana said, "Now! Jim will breathe better." At 10:15, the Lone Ranger and Tonto left while I stood in disbelief.

Diana called, took our phone calls and came over. She showed us how to adjust pillows, to modify his food, to increase his fluid, to keep track of his calories, to change the information in the daily notes. The health advice she gave us was invaluable, but what she did for me was miraculous. She instantly grasped the 'family dynamics,' and took the onus off me. With her help, I no longer felt like the interfering, inept, incompetent, pain of a family member. Diana was in charge. She said, "You folks got any problems. You write it in the log. This log is for me, and you tell them to me. Because this is about Jim's care!"

And later, when anyone complained, someone else would invariably write, "This is about Jim's care."

One afternoon, Carrie looked at me and said, "Diana has come down from heaven. She IS an angel." I never doubted it for a minute. Diana helped Jim and saved me.

If you live in the South long enough, sooner or later someone will say that someone has "been put in your path for a reason." Diana made adjustments to improve the quality of Jim's life and mine. In time, whenever there was a problem, the aides would say, "Why don't we ask Diana?"

Diana promised to be there when Jim died, but her career took her to the west coast. It would have been better for me had she been there, but I also knew that she would be better able to serve the greater good by working in the ACU of a hospital in Sacramento.

෧ ෳ

Diana had shifted the angle of Jim's bed to improve his breathing, so, you are damned if you do, … He slid down. We needed to lift Jim's ankles, because his left foot tended to swell. Did I say, damned if …? We tried a piece of old egg crate, sheepskin or pillow under his feet.

When Jim developed red marks on his toes and ankles, I bought sheepskin ankle protectors. Because the Velcro closing on the protectors irritated his skin, I bought a sheepskin bunny boot. To keep the blanket from rubbing on his feet, I bought a blanket lifter.

We worried he might fall out of bed. After searching for available products, I balked at paying close to $1,000 for a bed rail. Rick and Diana invented one out of PVC pipe (I am embarrassed to say I didn't pay for that; they did).

Initially, Jim had walked or run unaided and would tell Carrie, "I'm going to race you," and then he would take off. One day he had been sitting in a chair while Carrie walked the few steps into the kitchen. By the time she turned around he had gotten up, run to the end of the living room and fallen because he was unable to stop himself. Later he could walk by himself only with someone nearby. Still later he needed a hand on his elbow. I had bought him an elegant leather cane—another extravagant, dumb purchase. But Jim went from walking well, to walking badly, to a transport chair. He skipped 'cane' entirely. We got a gait belt to protect him. The blue belt – to match his eyes – was supposed to be around his waist, to ease him to the floor rather than have him fall uncontrollably and hurt himself. He resisted it, so it became the seat belt on his transport chair.

Jim rarely used the walker he got when he left the ACU, because he was too impaired to master it. I used it in the theatre when I played Grandma in *Tina and Tony's Wedding*. We needed the transport chair (Medicare paid for that). At first the chair I rented was simply in preparation for the hurricane season. Then we needed the chair all the time. He used it to go outside to sit by the water, to take out the garbage, to go to the bathroom, to the bedroom and into the kitchen for breakfast.

ৎ৵ ৵৶

If Jim fell, Carrie and Sylvia could lift him. The rest of us couldn't. One day, when Martha was taking him out of the shower, he said, "Oh, God, I am going down." She assured him he was safe. He said, "Thank God, I'm still alive."

I had installed grab bars near the toilet and in the shower stall, but he held the towel rack, which pulled away from the wall. A handyman replaced it and repainted that section of the wall. We removed the glass sliding shower doors and replaced them with a shower curtain and installed a handheld shower. We averaged three to five loads of laundry a day; we needed a new dryer.

We raised the level of the toilet with a commode. I bought a softer toilet seat – a waste of money. We bought a shower chair and a transfer bench – this time from a cancer thrift store for a $25 donation.

We bought wipes and latex-free, vinyl gloves by the case. We bought non-drying soaps, shampoos, moisturizers, wonder creams, moisture barrier creams, under neck creams, hydrocortisone ointments in various strengths, hemorrhoid suppositories, bag balm, talcum powders and cotton balls.

To prevent inflammation under his neck from Jim's relentless drooling, Diana suggested we use folded Kotex pads; however, I found soft burp cloths from a children's store; they were soft and worked like a charm. On some days the cloths needed to be changed every five minutes, so we needed pillow protectors.

Jim's swallowing deteriorated. No more finger foods like grapes and strawberries. We bought thickeners, nectars and cream soups. I bought a cup that came with a straw with a 'sort of' ball bearing in the bottom that caused the flow of liquid to slow. Then I found dysphagia cups, which he held himself. We had two – only $25 a piece. Frequently he offered his cup to Carrie, Sylvia or to me. I bought cutlery and cups for toddlers. Martha suggested we buy dishes with separators. I bought a blender for his protein drinks, a humidifier to keep his phlegm looser, and Vicks Vapo Rub and Eucalyptus Rub for his chest. We installed a new thermostat, because Diana suggested we keep the apartment cooler, and I bought a small Bose radio, so he could fall asleep listening to his music – extravagant, but music is what was left.

To prevent constipation, I bought Benefiber, Miralax, Milk of Magnesia and I bought Preparation H. Food was expensive. I don't mean the occasional Starbucks frappucino that he drank down in seconds. I mean the powdered protein and containers of Boost or Glycerna. Despite keeping a food log, with different people in the house, it was hard to know what foods were fresh. Did he eat half the soup yesterday or the day before? And everyone had a preference. "Please buy grits and sardines." "No, he likes oatmeal and banana." "Get him fruit". "He prefers coffee with cream," or "coffee without cream". "He likes maple syrup on his oatmeal". "He likes Amy's brand of pea soup." And I couldn't deprive him of his scallops or smoked salmon.

We needed laundry powder, fabric softener, stain remover, baking soda, Clorox, Lysol, Pine-Sol, big trash bags, and small ones for the wastebaskets.

With the spillage of drinks and medicine, Doug, the carpet cleaning man, came, but the kitchen rug was too stained to redeem. We were on a first-name basis with all the repairmen, including Cork-born Frank the plumber.

Later, we added no-rinse cloths for bed baths and a plastic basin. Jim got a fit of the giggles when Carrie washed him by putting the water in a wastepaper basket. We bought a remarkable contraption that fit under the top of the mattress, which worked on the principle of a vacuum and could lift him to a seated position.

∾ ∾

Besides listening to his coughing or hiccupping, at night I worried about money. What would we do if he outlived his long-term care insurance? How could I meet his expenses? Why had I gotten involved with theatre and wasted money? Could he become Medicaid-eligible? But Medicaid is about nursing homes, NOT home care. What would happen to me, if we used up our assets for his care?

I called our accountant, mildly hysterical, and asked, "What are we going to do? How do I prioritize our assets? Do I need a reverse mortgage? We are going through about $5,000 a month on his aides alone; our long-term care insurance will be gone by fall". Calmly, Michael said, "Let's talk at the end of the year."

While we had more money than some, we had less than others, and once he became ill, I worked only occasionally. Jim had taken a cut in pay when he accepted the chairman's job at HVCC, and even with an increase in salary with the promotion

to Dean, the move to HVCC affected his final average salary –
therefore, his pension, too. No regrets! Like the story of the
grasshopper and the ants, we had opted for the adventure. His
five years at the community college revitalized him. He had
implemented new courses, had recommended the theatre be
named for Maureen Stapleton, instituted an arts program,
established a jazz series, put art on the walls, and lived in his
beloved Columbia County. And living in Ireland was magic!

Like many other women, I had worked in several states in
different jobs that had or didn't have pension plans: 10 years in
New York City, three years in New Jersey, three years on
commission, five years in New York State and six in Ireland.

None of this was new to me. My father had gone through his
savings to pay for his 'minder.' My mother had a pension and
social security, but she too had a live-in caregiver, so in the end
she had her house, her pension and a small savings account.

When we bought the long-term care insurance, who would
have thought we would be dealing with a disease of
indeterminate length? While a five-year plan would have been
better, an unlimited policy would have been better still. At least
we had our three-year policy.

And no one knew Jim's life expectancy. One doctor
volunteered that Jim would die in two years. He didn't. Four
years later, he was alive. Another doctor said he would be in a
nursing home in six months. Three and a half years later, he was
still home. Someone said that I was taking too good care of him.
How does one respond to that? Apologize?

෴ ෴

Fortunately, we had wills, powers of attorney and advance
directives. Knowing he might have to become Medicaid-eligible,
early in his illness, when he still understood what he was
signing, we removed Jim's name from our joint assets and as the

beneficiary of my will. Then I took out a life insurance policy on myself to ensure Jim would have enough of his own money, if I died first. And I had heard that caregivers are statistically likely to die first.

There were ethical questions as well as financial ones. More than once his temperature was barely 0.6 degrees above normal; his legs wouldn't support him; he slept 24 hours, didn't eat or drink and had his first bed bath. I filled his standing prescription for Amoxicillin and realized how fragile his health was. *Would he survive without the antibiotic? Would the next bug kill him? Would Amoxicillin be enough? What are we fighting for? Has he had enough? Is he exhausted? Is this the quality of life he wanted? Is this the life that he wanted for both of us?* But when he smiled at me or at his food, or clapped his hands in the middle of watching a DVD, he was 'still there.'

What should I tell Ellen to do when it was my turn in the barrel? Keep me at home with help? Have enough saved to fly me to Amsterdam? Or Oregon? At what point would my health impact someone else's life or lives? Deplete someone else's resources? But parents are not spouses. It is the order of things for parents to die first. This was my husband not the annoying parent she had inherited by accident of birth.

My father had said, "Protect me from a long illness." I had been unable to do so because he had no notarized advance directives. All I could do was write a letter to the nursing home administrator explaining his wishes and sending a copy of a little card Dad kept in his wallet. Whenever my father developed pneumonia, he would be taken to the hospital, given an antibiotic and returned to the nursing home. While Jim and I had legal papers, they didn't tell me what to do. Was this the time to hold back the antibiotic, or was I making him more comfortable? Even when we signed our wills, we hadn't talked about death and dying. At least, I knew to get him a priest.

Not one member of our team of aides believed Jim would have lived as long if he had been in a nursing home.

At times he appeared close to death; at other times, he seemed as if he would live for years, so I needed to find out about Medicaid eligibility. I talked to eldercare attorneys – three in South Carolina, one in New York State and one in Massachusetts. Each state is different, and the system is complicated. At the time, every state permitted us to keep our primary residence, to have a car, and to fund our funeral arrangements. One lawyer suggested that we sell our assets, buy gold bars and put them into the walls of the apartment as decorations. In that way the gold would be part of our primary residence and untouchable by the government. "That will be $200, please."

When I asked another attorney about our Lenox condo, he advised me to get rid of it even though he had never been to the Berkshires. I said, "I am not ready to sell it, because I don't know where I am going to live when I lose Jim."

Another attorney in South Carolina wanted $17,000 in fees immediately to exploit a tax loophole that the governor was about to close. I was reminded of a banker who had said, "If someone needs an answer about money today, the answer is always 'No'." I didn't send the check and missed out on the loophole.

The attorney in Massachusetts explained that if Jim were put in a nursing home, and we couldn't pay the bill, then a lien would be put on our property. I could live in Lenox or repay the state when I sold the property. I hadn't a clue where I was going, so I did nothing.

A New York attorney told me to return to New York State as soon as Jim's insurance ran out, because "New York is more generous."

My classmate referred me to the director of a nursing home in New York City who said he would take Jim when I was ready.

To protect our assets, we would have had to simultaneously sell the condo in Hilton Head, the condo in Lenox, buy an apartment in New York, and air ambulance him to the facility – a logistical nightmare. What I learned was no matter how much I loved Jim – like so much else – the decisions would be about money. I was grateful that we had the coverage we had.

చ్ం ఆ

One day after bringing more groceries into the house and opening some UPS packages for Jim, I felt a wave of frustration. Like a petulant child, I wanted something for me, so I ordered a couple of books from the Quality Paperback Company.

Another time, I had been walking through the mall and could sense Jim beside me. I heard him say what he had said so often, "Buy something for yourself, Sweetie." I left without making a purchase. I couldn't think of anything I wanted or needed. And what difference did it make anyway?

But I wanted to spend some money on myself, not on him. I decided what I wanted was an expensive bar of soap. I don't recall whether it was Portuguese or French and whether it smelled of pear or banana, but I remember it cost almost $20, and the bar was so big it barely fit in the soap dish. But it was mine, and I put it in the bathroom that I used, that was almost mine.

చ్ం ఆ

Before we had help in the house, I had taken all my clothes from our bedroom closet and jammed them into the closet in the front bedroom, the computer room, the "supervisor's room." I could tiptoe out of the bedroom, shower and dress without waking him, which was important when he didn't sleep much. One morning I was standing in front of the mirror putting on my makeup, when I heard a god-awful roar like a lion. The sound was right next to me. I was so startled I grabbed my chest. I was terrified. Jim was standing in the doorway – roaring.

That scene might have been funny, but that roaring person did not seem amused. His eyes were wild. I tried to remain calm. I think I smiled and said, "Hi!" He didn't hurt me or continue roaring. He walked away, and I leaned over the sink and let out my breath. I had no idea why Jim roared.

Once we had help, however, the front room became the only space in the apartment that was mine. I came home one day to find one of the aides sitting on the sofa in the little room talking on my extension, so I asked if they all would consider that space off limits. They did.

The rest of the apartment was Jim's. Nothing was 'ours' or 'mine' anymore. I shared the house with Jim, the Roarer, and with his caregivers. The kitchen, the bathrooms, the living room, the bedroom were theirs. I had virtually no privacy unless it was in the middle of the night and Jim was asleep. The dishes, the drawers, the cupboards were no longer just ours, even the newspapers. One Sunday morning, I was asked, "Where's Jim's paper?" *Jim's paper.* A friend came by one day and sat on the porch with me for a few minutes. She looked around at the view, at the apartment, at Jim, at the women caring for him, and said, "What a beautiful prison!"

Jim had talked to me at the same time I was on the phone; later, because I was so rarely alone, it was difficult to have a private conversation, though the aides did their best to give me some privacy when I needed it. And when the phone rang, and I answered, it usually wasn't for me. My toilet, my toilet paper, refrigerator, husband, TV, washer, dryer were communal. It was like living in a dorm.

One evening when Sylvia had gone, and Jim was asleep, I stretched out on the sofa in the living room and luxuriated in the moment. I was alone with Jim. It was quiet and peaceful, and no one was being blamed for anything. Heaven! Jim was the patient, the focus of their attention, and I was either interfering or irrelevant. I had wanted him home – but I didn't have a home of my own any more, and that was part of the price I paid.

Late in Jim's illness, I reclaimed the front room, and gave up the car as my private space, the place I had used to talk on my cell phone, open the mail, cry or scream, write checks, pay my bills, and learn lines. I came home. I stopped going to Starbucks or Barnes & Noble to read or write. I filed papers again. I gave up having someone else file medical insurance. I even bought a little TV. I closed the door.

೫ ೭

Another cost of Jim's illness was people. As Jim changed, the people who had known him before he became sick changed too. Friends couldn't cope with his condition. True, Jim was not pretty to look at. His lower lip was slack. He was bent over, his eyes were less focused, his tremors more pronounced, his drooling constant and his hands never still.

But he always appeared to enjoy a friendly face, some 'conversation' and a handshake. A neighbor said, "We don't want to see him like this." Another old friend said, "It's too hard for me." Someone else asked, "Is he better?"

And people said remarkable things: "You should never have married an older man." Someone in our building said, "This isn't a nursing home." I heard the classic, "God only gives you what you can handle." All I wanted to hear was, "How are you? How is Jim?" One old friend did come over; she dropped by to say, "Hello," to smile and to wait for him to smile back.

If you were a social worker, physical therapist, doctor, aide or a nurse with a hard edge, he might not welcome you pleasantly. If you were there to fix the air conditioning or the toilet, if you were the plumber with the friendly smile and a great

handshake, or the neighbor who said, "How are you doing?",
Jim would muster a wonderful smile and say, "Still working" or
"I'm retired."

∽ ∾

When Father McCaffrey retired, I had gone to see another priest,
who recommended I read Rabbi Kushner's book, *When Bad
Things Happen to Good People*. Father West was a bright young
priest with a huge parish. Despite his commitments, he came by
to see Jim. He knelt by his chair. Jim was focused on the Land's
End catalog he was shredding and didn't look up. When he
finally did, he smiled at Father West who had deliberately worn
his collar. Jim seemed happy to see this stranger. Father West
spoke about having visited Ireland and then blessed Jim and
recited *The Lord's Prayer*. Jim's eyes closed. Who knows why?
But after Father West left, Jim began to 'sing.' It went something
like "doo, doo, doo, doo."

Jack Brennan, a retired physician, would see me in the
parking lot and ask, "Is there anything I can do?" I always said,
"I wish." He asked if he could come over and visit. He did. He
sat with Jim and held his hand, while Jim muttered
unintelligibly and incomprehensibly. Jack hung on Jim's
indecipherable words. Before he left, Jack looked at me and said,
"This means more to me than it does to him. Thank you for
letting me come up."

∽ ∾

Jim died on January 6, 2006, officially at 10:15 am. His skin
looked jaundiced, and he emitted an ugly gag. No Hollywood
death this. Dr. Brennan saw the horror on my face and said, "Jim
is already gone. It is his body's last gasp." It was over. Jim was
no more except in my memory and in my heart.

His final days began on Christmas Eve. The women had left early because of the holiday. Jim was sitting up in bed. I had defrosted a favorite dish: lobster wrapped in sole. I fed him and went back into the kitchen to clean up. When I came back into the bedroom, I saw he was drooling black liquid. Despite the fact that it was Christmas Eve, I had taken Jack Brennan at his word and phoned him. He came right over and explained that it was bile. I asked him what I could do. He said, "Jim's system is breaking down." I still didn't get it. Jim was peaceful. Dr. Brennan left and said he would be back in the morning, Christmas Day.

I cleaned Jim up, and we lay down to rest. As so often before, I was half awake through the night. But there was no repeat. Dr. Brennan came back in the morning, but Jim no longer wanted food. When we put a spoon to his lips, his mouth stayed closed. His eyes were closed too.

Dr. Brennan called our internist, and they arranged for a hospice nurse to come in – a different hospice.

However, there was miscommunication, and a nurse from the home health division came over instead of from hospice. Because Jim had not eaten anything since the lobster, I asked if we could give him some fluid with an IV. We did.

Jim had one IV. Later that afternoon, he opened his eyes, smiled and began to twist the dial of his little portable radio. We were so excited. I remember calling Carrie on her cell saying, "He's back."

But it wasn't to be. The nurse from home health said, "Now he needs to take fluid on his own. Every 15 minutes give him some fluid." Jim slept through the night. Now barely wakening in the morning, there were to be no more IVs. "Come on, Jim."

When one of the aides arrived the next morning, she looked angry. She had talked to another aide and they were considering taking Jim to a hospital, because they thought I was killing him. I was stunned. The next day I showed her our advance directives.

I showed her the date, 1993, and Jim's signature. I said, "I probably shouldn't have even given him the first IV."

After that remark I kept it together long enough to say, "It is your job to get fluids down Jim every 15 minutes. I am going to the supermarket to buy consommé, ice pops and Jello." I raced down the stairs, a scream in my throat. My husband was dying, and one of his caregivers thought I was killing him. Thankfully, I bumped into Dr. Brennan as I was running to my car. I didn't even say, "Good morning." I looked at him and blurted out what had just been said to me. He advised me to try not to take what had been said to heart.

Somehow, I drove to the supermarket. I don't remember but, once there, the enormity of what was happening, Jim's dying, and my shock at what had been said, it all hit me. I wept as I grabbed the items I was looking for. A young woman who was stocking the shelves asked, "What's wrong?" I told her. I don't remember her name, but I do remember her putting her arm around my shoulders and comforting me.

I was touched – deeply touched. I paid and raced back home. I asked how he was doing. I tried to give him liquid myself – with a dropper. I tried the soup, the ice pops, nothing. His lips stayed closed; his eyes stayed closed. Was there any cognition? Was he saying, "No more, I have had enough?" Part of me was hoping that he not I was making the decision. I was hoping that he was giving up the struggle because he was too tired to go on any more.

I don't remember whether it was that day or the next when we stopped trying to give him fluids. The nurses from hospice dropped by. Unbelievably, one asked if we thought he had 'food poisoning.' Nine years of loving him, caring for him, making sure he was safe, and now I was being asked if the lobster wrapped in sole had killed him. *Dear God!*

The days went by. Jim slept. I pushed the twin beds together and lay by his side and held his hand and listened to his breathing – the long silences followed by normal breaths, the warmth of his hand in mine, the softness of his skin.

Jim was dying. The dawning, the disbelief, the realization that this time he was, in fact, dying. No Amoxicillin could save him. The women were there. They took turns staying through the night. One night we all slept on the floor. They rolled him, changed him, and gave him a bed bath. He never opened his eyes. Father West came by on January 5 in the evening to sit with me. He went into the bedroom and spoke to Jim and told him to, "Let go." I kept the CD player on by his bedside and played Brahms' *German Requiem*, Vivaldi, and something by Yo-Yo Ma.

Ten days after the bile oozed from his lips, the men from the funeral home came with their gurney to take his body away. I kissed him one more time and said to now deaf ears, "Thank you, Cookie."

ﷺ ﷺ

I have little recollection of what happened next. I must have hugged Dr. Brennan, the hospice nurse and Denise. I am sure it was Denise who told me to call the funeral home. I called Kevin and Ellen. I had phoned them both earlier in the week once I knew Jim wasn't having another IV and wasn't taking any fluids. That morning I reached Kevin at work and told him his father had died and that I would let him know when the funeral Mass would be. I have no idea how I said it. Nor do I remember what I said to Ellen other than to tell her Jim had died and to please find a way to come.

Numb? Mechanical? Disassociated? I was going through the motions. I was doing what I was supposed to do.

Despite the people who were still in the apartment, I remember the emptiness, the absence, the void, the loneliness.

The whole apartment had breathed in and was holding its breath. Everything changed with Jim's last breath.

There were no tears now; perhaps I was too stunned. And yet how could I be stunned, when he had been dying for years and 'actively dying' for 10 days. There could be no 'ambivalence' anymore. Jim was dead.

It was over. And I hoped that somewhere in his profoundly damaged brain, he knew how much I loved him, how much our lives together had meant to me. And how profoundly I would continue to miss him. I hoped he knew that I tried to be there for him. He once said, "Dignity matters so much to you." I hope he knew how I had tried to maintain his dignity, lamely, but I had tried to protect him.

We had never been able to say, "Good-bye." There was never going to be some exquisite deathbed aphorism from Jim. I remember the hollowness. With all my heart, I hoped he had heard Father West and had chosen to "let go." After the obligatory phone calls, I walked back into the living room.

A well-intentioned hospice nurse placed Jim's photograph on a side table between us, sat down, looked at me and said, "So tell me, how did you two meet?"

EPILOGUE

Everywhere, we learn only from those whom we love.

Goethe

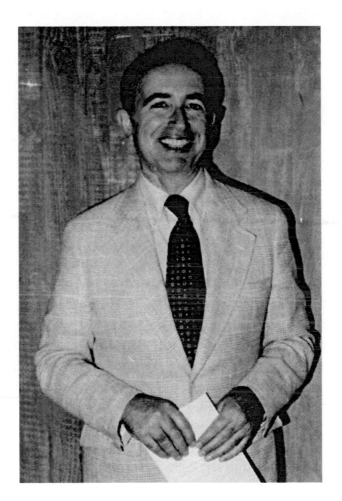

It's been more than five years since Jim died. I live in the Berkshires now, and I have another cat. He is Jack, named for Jim's favorite uncle, Jack, Jim's favorite Irish artist, Jack Yeats, and for Jack McCoy on *Law and Order*.

Since Jim's death, I have roamed about in search of home: Portland, Oregon and New York City. I taught in Spain for a couple of semesters. Jack came with me. I miss Jim profoundly. I suppose the only difference from now and then is that I remember more of the healthy times than the sick ones. For sure, I am not as light-hearted or funny as I used to be, but fortunately I see more of the happy images than the cruel ones, but I can't delete them from my memory bank. I still wonder why we got this 'bad hand.' If Jim were around, he probably could 'spin' it for me.

I remember with profound gratitude the people who were there for him and for me and with deep disappointment the ones who weren't or who couldn't be – and members of the healthcare community are in both groups. I tend to give Western medicine a wide berth now and seek alternative approaches; but if doctors, nurses and aides remember that warmth and listening are essential to quality care – even if they cannot cure – perhaps my faith in my dad's profession will be restored.

I hope the statistics about dementia are wrong and that the researchers find a way to beat these diseases, because more often than not, dementia affects our elders, the historical memory of our society – our collective wisdom. On a more personal level, I hope I made more right choices than wrong ones for Jim and for me. But it's over, and now it's about putting one foot in front of the other and trying to find purpose and meaning.

My heart goes out to anyone and everyone who is a caregiver, with special empathy for those facing the horror of dementia. To paraphrase Jim, "You'll get through this." Just be gentle on yourselves. As he wrote, "One must be content to be happy in small ways."

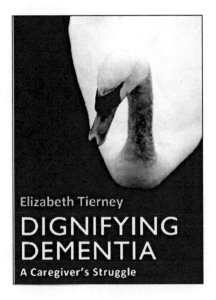

Elizabeth Tierney

DIGNIFYING DEMENTIA

A Caregiver's Struggle

If you would like to share your comments and reactions on *Dignifying Dementia,* you can do so at **www.dignifyingdementia.com.**

I hope that, in time, the website will become a valuable resource of shared experiences and knowledge for anyone who is caregiving for someone they love who suffers from dementia.

ACKNOWLEDGEMENTS

This book would have remained some pages in a box and never have seen the light of day had it not been for Rae Eastman's belief in its merit. And then it might have remained an undeleted file on my computer had it not been for publisher Brian O'Kane and his team at Oak Tree Press: Rita, Anne and Andrea. I thank them all for their patience, insight, sensitivity and commitment.

Thank you to them, and to Jim's devoted caregivers, compassionate doctors and nurses, patient friends, concerned family members, sensitive neighbors, generous members of the clergy and complete strangers who were there for him and for me during his illness.

There are no words to express my gratitude for all their kindness.

ABOUT THE AUTHOR

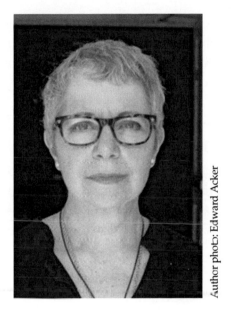

Author photo: Edward Acker

Elizabeth P. Tierney, Ph.D. is a writer, trainer, consultant and lecturer in Communications and Management. She was a school administrator in the US and taught at University College Dublin, Ireland and at Cesuga in Spain. She has trained and coached students and business people, spoken at conferences and is the author of seven books, including two published by Oak Tree Press: *Show Time!* and *Selling Yourself.*

ABOUT OAK TREE PRESS

Oak Tree Press develops and delivers information, advice and resources for entrepreneurs and managers. It is Ireland's leading business book publisher, with an unrivalled reputation for quality titles across business, management, HR, law, marketing and enterprise topics. NuBooks is its recently-launched imprint, publishing short, focused ebooks for busy entrepreneurs and managers.

In addition, through its founder and managing director, Brian O'Kane, Oak Tree Press occupies a unique position in start-up and small business support in Ireland through its standard-setting titles, as well training courses, mentoring and advisory services.

Oak Tree Press is comfortable across a range of communication media – print, web and training, focusing always on the effective communication of business information.

Oak Tree Press, 19 Rutland Street, Cork, Ireland.

T: + 353 21 4313855 F: + 353 21 4313496.

E: info@oaktreepress.com W: www.oaktreepress.com.